HEART CARE

ISBN: 81-7436-118-9

Lustre Press Pvt. Ltd.
M-75 Greater Kailash II (Market)
New Delhi 110 048, India
Phones: (011) 6442271, 6462782, 6460886
Fax: (011) 6467185, E-mail: roli@vsnl.com
Website: rolibooks.com

Text: Dr (Prof) H.S. Wasir
Graphic Illustrations: Jai Kumar Sharma
Photographs: Dheeraj Paul, Manisha Gera Baswani

Printed and bound in Singapore

HEART CARE

for Holistic Health

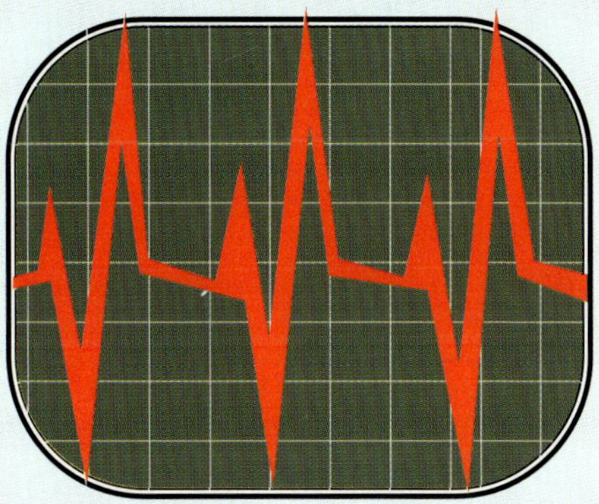

DR (PROF) H.S. WASIR

M.D., D.M., F.A.M.S., F.I.M.S.A.,F.N.A.Sc.

Lustre Press

Roli Books

He who wishes to protect from harm this great organ-the heart, those great rooted ones – the coronary blood vessels, and the vital essence, should scrupulously avoid all that causes affliction to the mind.

—Charaka Samhita

Contents

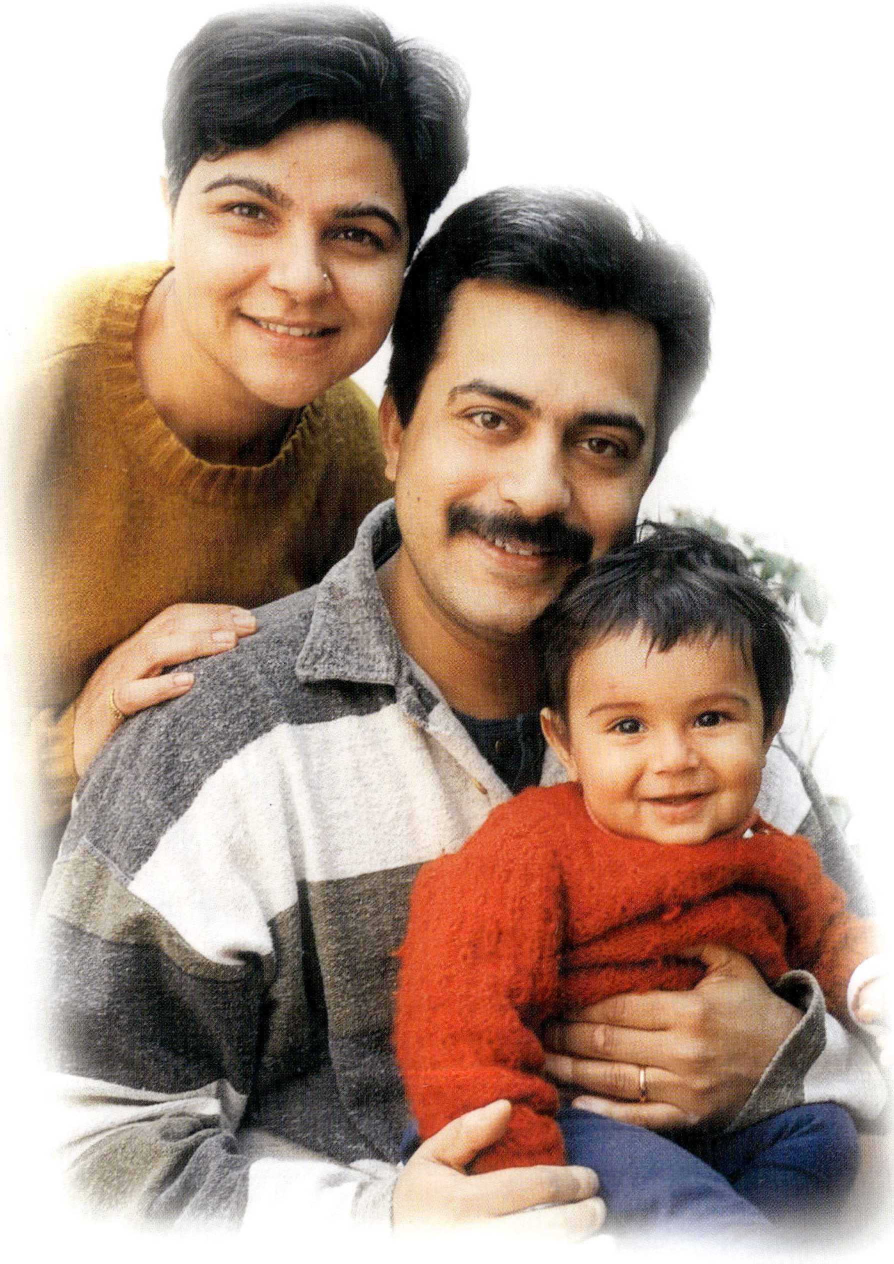

1. Healthy Living for a Healthy Heart

There is a close symbiotic link between leading a healthy lifestyle and the well-being of the heart. Conversely, if anything goes wrong with the heart, there is an adverse effect on the whole body which is manifested through one or more of the cardinal symptoms of heart disease such as palpitation, breathlessness, fatigue, chest pain or blackouts. Keeping the body disease free indicates positive health, while negative health denotes the presence of disease. The heart is a tough organ supplying nutrition to the whole body, but it does need nourishment for its own well-being also.

Food for the heart consists mainly of three 'dishes': **A Balanced Diet** containing desirable amounts of proteins, carbohydrates, fats, vitamins and minerals like potassium, sodium, magnesium and calcium; **Regular Physical Exercise** and **Mental Relaxation** through meditation, prayer and yoga. This, in turn, helps in avoiding undue and harmful fluctuations in heart rhythm and blood pressure in response to the stressful challenges of the environment. The 'salad' and 'spices' that enhance the food value for the positive health of the heart and the body come from one's character (*aachaar*), thinking process (*vichaar*) and interpersonal dealings (*vyavhaar*). The role of all these aspects in positive health is of equal importance. The food we eat, the water we drink and the air we breathe play a significant role in human health, prevention of disease and preservation of life at the optimum level. The factors that cause a negative turnabout in positive health are habits such as sedentary living, cigarette smoking, addiction to drugs and alcohol and a hostile environment. In fact, an increasingly distressing factor is that more and more people in their thirties and forties are prone to sudden heart attack.

The heart is the only organ in the body which works non stop like a sentinel on duty (see overleaf). Although modern drugs, surgical intervention and invasive devices are providing a new lease of life to more and more people, they can only be 'full of life' if they focus on healthy living.

THE HUMAN HEART

The nucleus of the cardiovascular system is the heart. Blood is pumped to and from the heart in a figure of eight path through two circuits of blood vessels. The right side of the heart receives oxygen-poor blood from the whole body and pumps this blood to the lungs for oxygenation through the pulmonary artery. The oxygen-rich blood is returned to the left side of the heart via the pulmonary veins. The aorta, the body's largest artery, supplies the body's organs with oxygen-pure blood. From these organs veins merge to form the superior vena cava and inferior vena cava, which empty oxygen-poor blood to the right side of the heart for recirculation through the lungs.

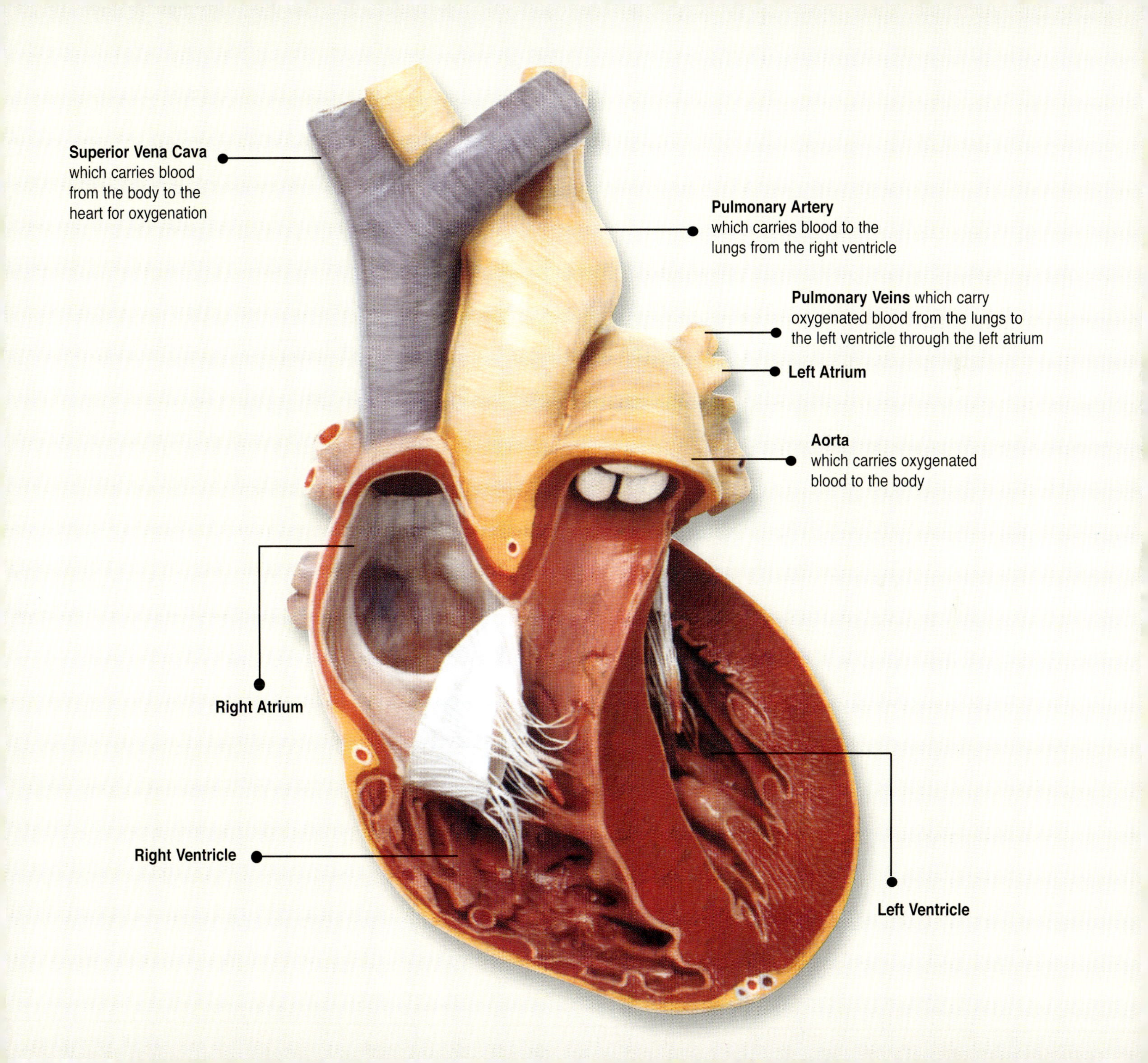
Superior Vena Cava which carries blood from the body to the heart for oxygenation
Pulmonary Artery which carries blood to the lungs from the right ventricle
Pulmonary Veins which carry oxygenated blood from the lungs to the left ventricle through the left atrium
Left Atrium
Aorta which carries oxygenated blood to the body
Right Atrium
Right Ventricle
Left Ventricle

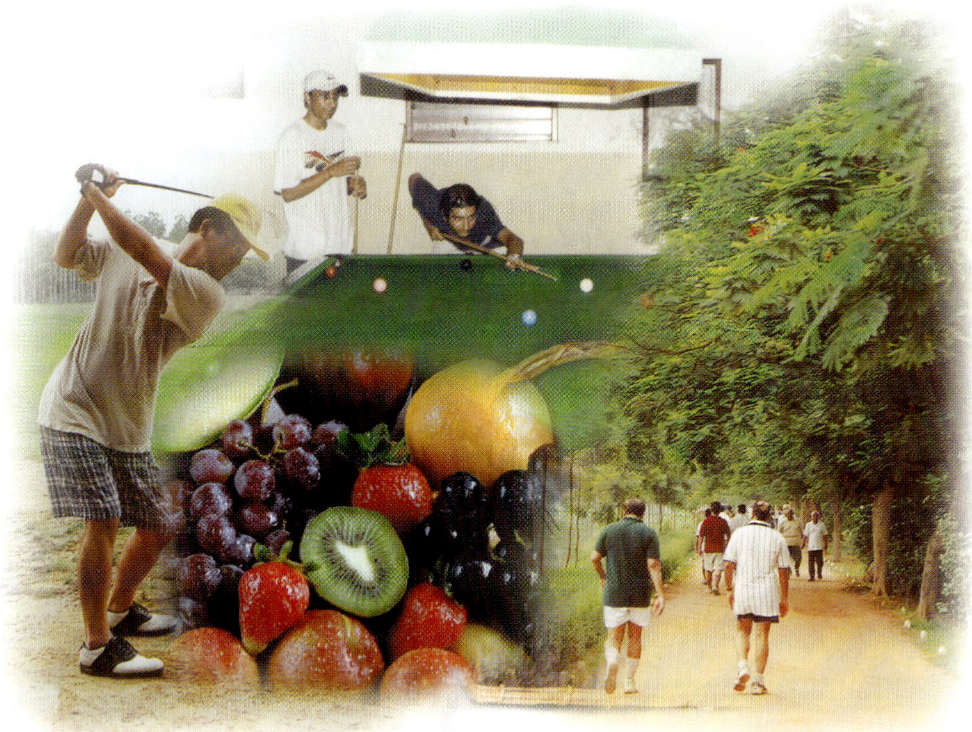

2. Leading a Balanced Lifestyle

Human longevity and good health are affected by one's lifestyle. Controlling, preventing and eradicating faulty habits can reduce and remove morbidity and ensure a productive life.

Overeating – An Obese Problem

Obesity has a direct relationship with disease, disability and death. Central obesity — when the waist is bigger than the hips — is a risk factor for heart attacks. Except for a rare instance when an obese individual may enjoy good health into old age, generally, obesity is inversely proportional to long life.

Cutting Down on Cholesterol

As the weight rises, the cholesterol also rises, and this equation is, by and large, diet related. The 'good' or 'friendly' cholesterol called HDL (High Density Lipoprotein), comes down as the body weight goes up. We should, therefore, eat foods which do not increase bad

STANDARD HEIGHT & WEIGHT FOR MEN AND WOMEN

Height		Standard Weight: Man		Standard Weight: Woman	
CM	FT	KG	LBS	KG	LBS
152.2	5'-0"			50.8-54.4	112-120
154.8	5'-1"			51.7-55.3	114-122
157.3	5'-2"	56.3-60.3	124-133	53.1-56.7	117-125
159.8	5'-3"	57.6-61.7	127-136	54.4-58.1	120-128
162.4	5'-4"	58.9-63.5	130-140	56.3-59.9	124-132
164.9	5'-5"	60.8-65.3	134-144	57.6-61.2	127-135
167.5	5'-6"	62.2-66.7	137-147	58.9-63.5	130-140
170.0	5'-7"	64.0-68.5	141-151	60.8-65.3	134-144
172.5	5'-8"	65.8-70.8	145-156	62.2-66.7	137-147
175.1	5'-9"	67.6-72.6	149-160	64.0-68.5	141-151
177.6	5'-10"	69.4-74.4	153-164	65.8-70.3	145-155
180.2	5'-11"	71.2-76.2	157-168	67.1-71.7	148-158
182.7	6'-0"	73.0-78.5	161-173	68.5-73.9	151-163
185.2	6'-1"	75.3-80.7	166-178	–	–
187.8	6'-2"	77.6-83.5	171-184	–	–
190.3	6'-3"	79.8-85.7	176-189	–	–

CHOLESTEROL CONTENT OF VARIOUS FOODS

Food	Quantity (g)	Household Measure	Cholesterol Content (mg)
Meat & its products			
Hen egg (yellow)	100 g	2	420
Chicken (broiler)	100 g	1 portion	60
Mutton (goat) (Medium fat lean)	100 g	3-4 pieces	65
Liver	100 g	4-6 pieces	300
Kidney	100 g	2 pieces	150
Brain	100 g	7 tbsp	250
Pork	100 g	1 slice	70
Oysters	100 g	1 portion	230-47 mg
Shrimps	100 g	1 portion	150 mg
Crab	100 g	1 portion	145 mg
Pork ribs	100 g	2	105 mg
Lamb	100 g	1 portion	70 mg
Milk & its products			
Whole milk	100 ml	1 small cup	11
Skimmed milk	100 ml	1 small cup	2.4
Cream	100 ml	1 small cup	100
Butter	100 g	1 small cup	240
Cheese	100 g	4 slices	16
Ice cream plain	100 g	1 small cup	375
Animal fat	100 g	1 small cup	90

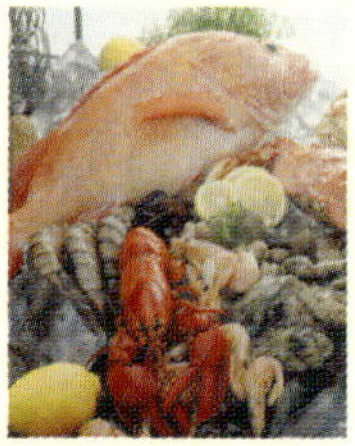

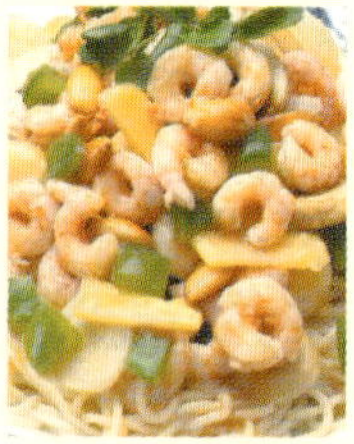

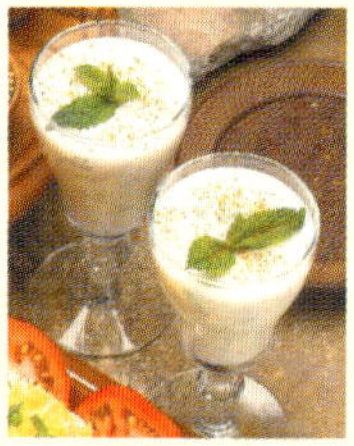

Source: *Nutritive Value of Indian Foods,* National Institute of Nutrition, Hyderabad, India.

FOODS RICH IN CHOLESTEROL

Meat and its products
Hen egg (yellow), liver, kidney, oysters, shrimps, crab, pork ribs, pork, lamb, mutton (goat)

Milk and its products
Ice cream, butter, cream, animal fat

FOOD WITH NO CHOLESTEROL

Cereals and pulses, vegetables, fruits, dry fruits & nuts

Source: *Nutritive Value of Indian Foods,* National Institute of Nutrition, Hyderabad, India.

cholesterol (LDL-Low Density Lipoprotein) and lower the HDL since the HDL is a protective factor against heart attacks. The dietary source of cholesterol is food of animal origin such as milk, dairy products and meat.

Cumulative data of various studies from several countries shows that as the cholesterol levels increase, so do the trends of mortality due to cardiovascular disease. And if we add smoking to obesity, then this adds fuel to the fire, thus further increasing mortality and morbidity, especially due to cardiovascular diseases in both males and females.

There is enough evidence to show that overweight shortens the lifespan, and overweight is usually caused by overeating and eating calorie-rich foods such as sweets and fried foodstuff. We must, therefore, attack the problem at its roots by restricting food intake to avoid becoming fat. Losing weight through high-cost slimming centres is only a temporary achievement. Permanent weight control can only be attained by consuming a low-calorie, balanced vitamin-protein diet supplemented by regular physical exercise.

INTERRELATIONSHIP BETWEEN DIET AND OTHER RISK FACTORS

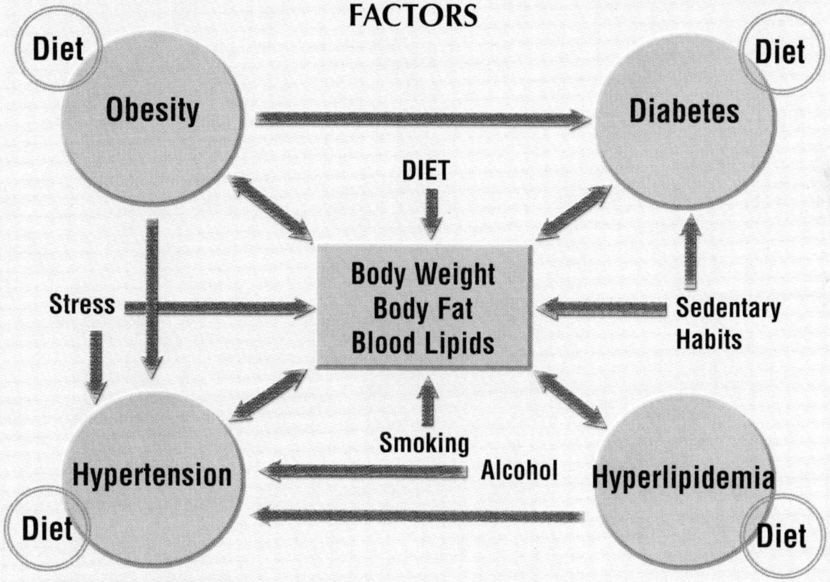

Necessary Nutrition

An American physician named Dean Ornish wrote a book on reversal of atherosclerosis. He stated that if the diet was changed from non-vegetarian to vegetarian and regular physical exercise, yoga and meditation were incorporated, atherosclerosis — the narrowing of partially blocked arteries — could be reversed. Food for the heart comprises: (1) a balanced diet containing high fibre, complex carbohydrates like tubers and roots; (2) regular physical exercise and (3) a relaxed mind. This is the tripod of longevity. While a vegetarian diet

CIRCULATION OF BLOOD

The right side of the heart receives blood from the veins and pumps it to both the lungs where it is oxygenated. The left side of the heart receives the oxygenated blood from the lungs and pumps it through the aorta to the rest of the body.

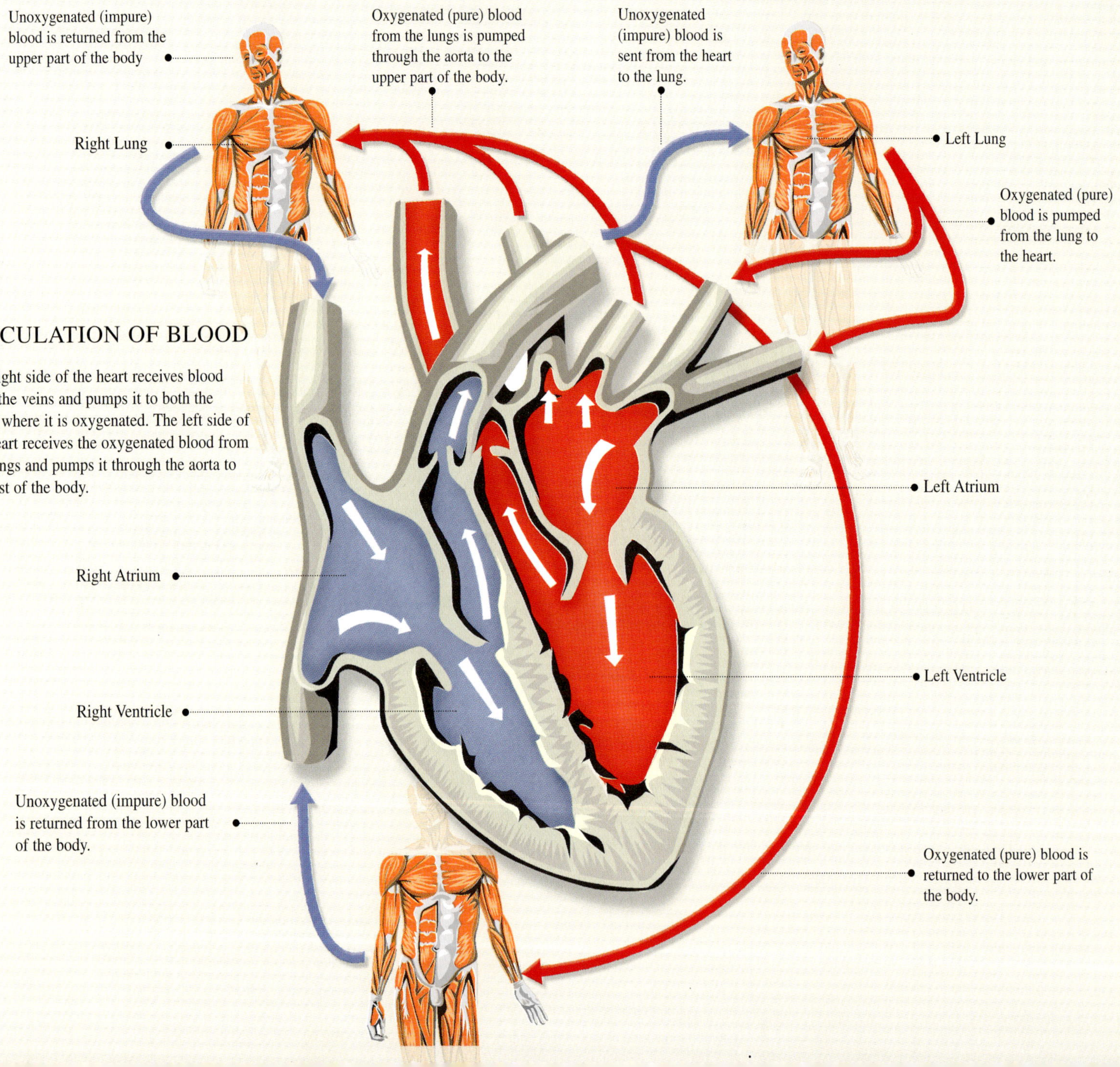

CIRCULATION OF BLOOD

Blood flows in a continuous stream even when the heart relaxes between contractions. Arteries have thick walls so that they can sustain the high pressure created when the heart pumps blood through them. The arteries expand and then recoil to push the blood forward. Veins have thinner walls than the arteries because the blood flowing through them flows at a lower pressure. Veins contain valves which prevent the backflow of blood away from the heart. Capillaries are the smallest blood vessels through which food and oxygen pass into the tissue fluid and, in return, waste is carried in the reverse direction.

HIGH POTASSIUM FOODS*

Name of Food	Potassium (mg/100 g)
Whole Bengal gram (*chana*)	808
Split Bengal gram (*chana dal*)	720
Whole black gram (*sabut urad*)	800
Black-eyed peas (*lobia*)	1132
Whole green gram (*sabut moong*)	844
Moth beans (*moth*)	1096
Split green gram (*moong dal*)	1160
Split red gram (*arhar dal*)	1104
Peas, dry (*mattar*)	724
Spinach (*palak*)	206
Colocasia (*arbi*)	280
Sweet potato (*shakarkand*)	500
Apricots (*khoomani*)	430
Fresh sweet lime (*musambi*)	490
Peaches (*arroo*)	453
Plums (*alu bokhara*)	247
Milk (buffalo)	140
Yoghurt	260

*Foods which help in lowering high blood pressure.
Source: *Nutritive Value of Indian Foods.* National Institute of Nutrition, Hyderabad, India, 1990.

does not provide permanent immunity from heart attacks, consuming meat in moderation, specially white meat and fish, along with the usual quota of vegetables and fruits may not be harmful for health in general and the heart in particular. If the uric acid and blood cholesterol levels are normal, a mixed non-vegetarian and vegetarian diet (omnivorous habit) is better for a healthy heart.

It is a common saying that we become what we eat. Foods that protect against heart attacks, high blood pressure, stroke and cancer — the main modern killers — are vegetables, whole fruits, coarse grains and bread made from coarse ground flour. Milk and yoghurt should be taken in moderation and extra salt and excess alcohol should be avoided. A diet rich in potassium (fresh whole fruits, vegetables and nuts) and low in sodium (avoid preserved foods and pickles) is helpful in the prevention of hypertension and stroke.

Staying Physically Fit

Along with a balanced diet, physical exercise plays an important role in

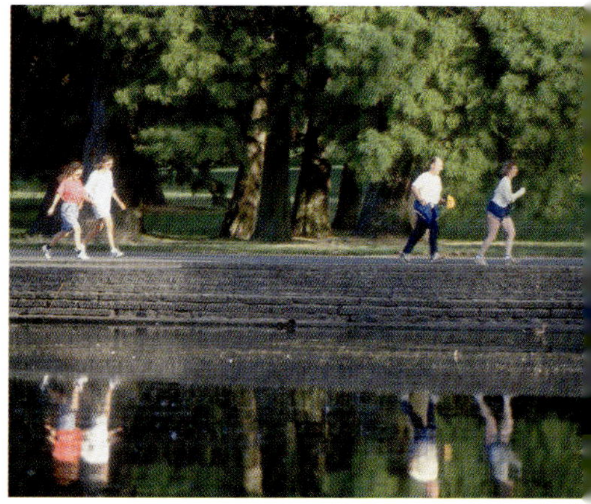

achieving a long and healthy life. We know that physically active populations have a higher longevity than physically inactive or sedentary ones. Fitness needs vary and one must cater to them individually.

Avoiding Excessive Alcohol

Alcohol intake probably dates back to time immemorial, as its descriptions are available in ancient texts both in India and abroad. It is well known that heart attacks are less common in those populations that consume moderate amounts of alcohol. Wine consumption (fermented alcohol) is, perhaps, more cardio-protective than distilled alcohol as appears from observing the French who have fewer cases of coronary disease compared to UK and other countries where whisky consumption is more prevalent. Excessive alcohol consumption (more than two ounces a day) results in major medical problems including alcoholism (addiction), liver cirrhosis, cognitive and neurological disorders, accidents, hypertension, arrhythmias, stroke, increased overall mortality and

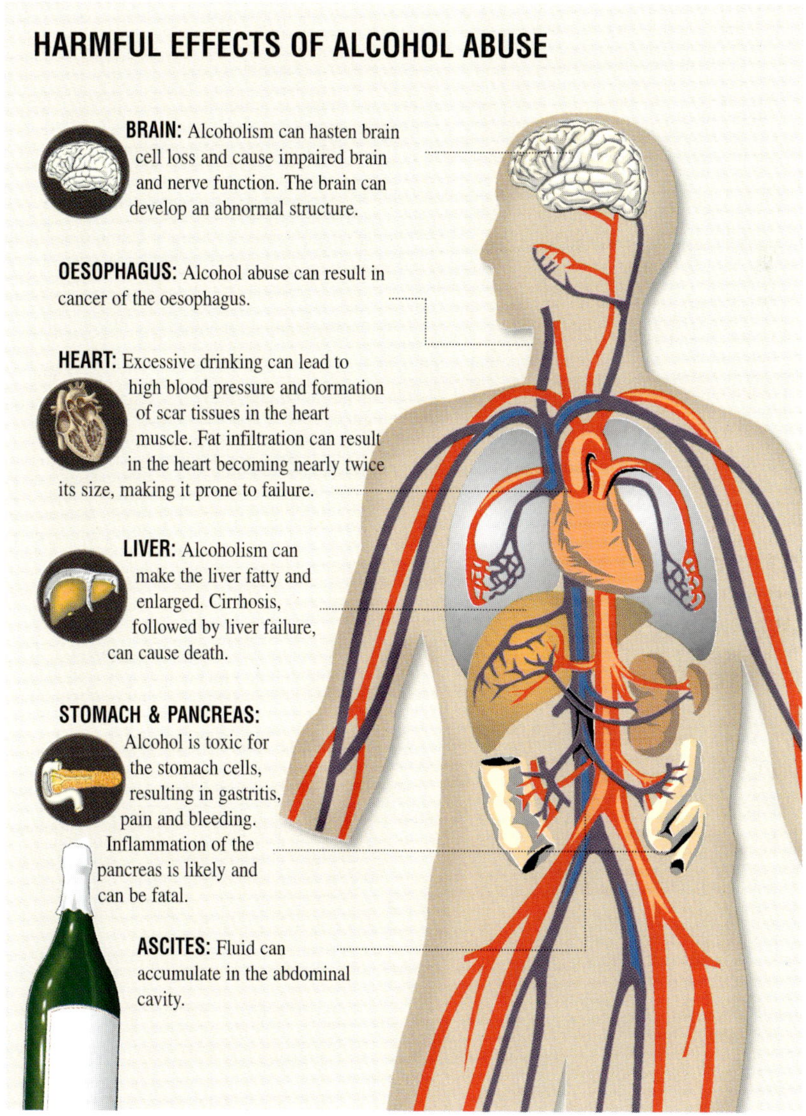

defects in babies whose mothers drink alcohol during pregnancy.

Although a small amount of alcohol consumption may be beneficial for prevention of coronary artery disease and improving social interaction, yet the harmful medical, social and economic effects of alcohol abuse clearly outweigh its cardio-protective effects. It has been estimated that the overall damages of alcohol misuse such as health-related disorders, social problems, accidents, divorces and imprisonment are greater than those due to smoking and use of illicit drugs.

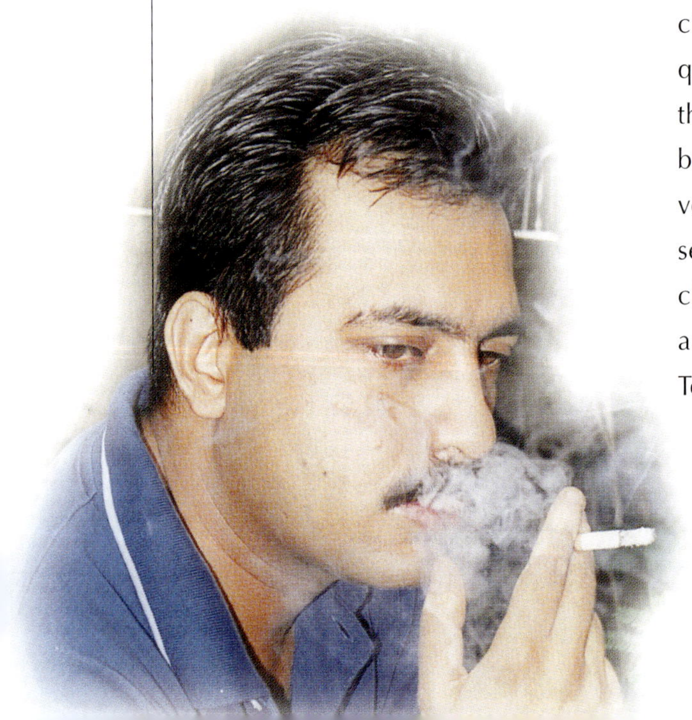

Shunning Smoking

Smoking decreases longevity and the decrease in lifespan is directly proportionate to the number of cigarettes smoked per day. The quality of life is adversely affected by the occurrence of diseases like bronchitis, angina and hoarseness of voice. Smoking also decreases sexual potency and causes claudication (cramping pain due to arterial obstruction) of the legs. Tobacco consumption is a major cause of death and disability both in developed and developing countries — more so now in the latter.

CALORIFIC VALUE OF HARD AND SOFT DRINKS

	Quantity	Calories (K cal)
Beer	250 ml	122
Brandy	30 ml	98
Gin	30 ml	84
Rum	30 ml	98
Whisky	30 ml	91
Champagne (dry)	100 ml	78
Red wine	100 ml	82
White wine	100 ml	75
Sherry	30 ml	43
Port	30 ml	51
Cola	1 bottle	84
Orange drink	1 bottle	84
Lemon drink	1 bottle	84
Plain soda	1 bottle	0

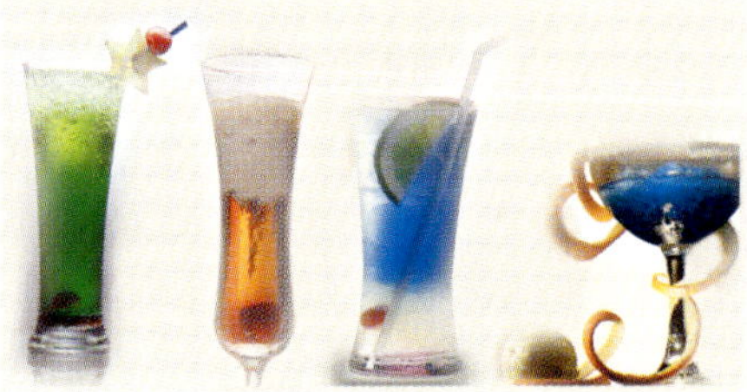

Dos	Don'ts
❑ Exercise at least four times a week. ❑ Walk or cycle short distances instead of taking a car. ❑ Take the stairs up to a few floors. Say NO to the lift. ❑ Eat salads and vegetables with every meal. ❑ Take that occasional vacation.	❑ Don't sleep that extra hour. ❑ Avoid smoking. ❑ Don't drink too much too often. ❑ Don't gorge on desserts and fried foods. ❑ Don't skip meals.

Not only does smoking adversely affect the smoker, but those who happen to be in the vicinity of the smoker also bear its brunt as passive smokers by inhaling 'second hand' smoke. Smoking during pregnancy results in low birth weight of the yet-to-be-born, premature births and spontaneous abortions.

The list of diseases that results from tobacco consumption is a rather lengthy one and includes:

1. Lung diseases like bronchitis and lung cancer
2. Heart diseases like heart attacks
3. Diseases of the blood vessels like hardening of the arteries which results in a diminished blood supply to the limbs, causing pain in the legs on walking
4. Cancer of the oral cavity (like the tongue and the mouth), voice-box and the urinary bladder
5. Defects in the foetus and newborn babies of smoking mothers
6. Impotence and impaired libido due to atherosclerosis of the blood vessels supplying the genitalia

Mental Relaxation

Stress and emotions have two aspects — the physiological and the psychological. Under a stressful situation, there is a rise in pulse rate, an increase in oxygen demand by the tissues and an increase in cardiac output.

There are two types of emotions: positive and negative. Negative emotions give rise to stress. Desires, worry, anger and attachment to worldly pleasures result in an increase of heart rate, blood pressure (see p. 41) and rate pressure product (heart rate x systolic pressure). It is this double product (rate pressure product), which is important for the oxygen requirement by the heart and, hence, the patient suffers when harbouring negative emotions. On the other hand, positive emotions like selfless service, giving without expecting in return, and a 'May-I-Help-You' attitude result in peace, tranquillity and equilibrium of self. Positive emotions keep the blood pressure and heart rate under desirable control, thereby protecting the heart and cardiovascular system against the adverse effects that are produced with negative emotions.

Yoga for a Tranquil Mind: There are various ways in which one can achieve mental relaxation. One of the best ways is through YOGA. In yoga there are exercises or body positions called *asanas* which open the energy channels in the body. Practising *asanas* helps the body to develop steadiness.

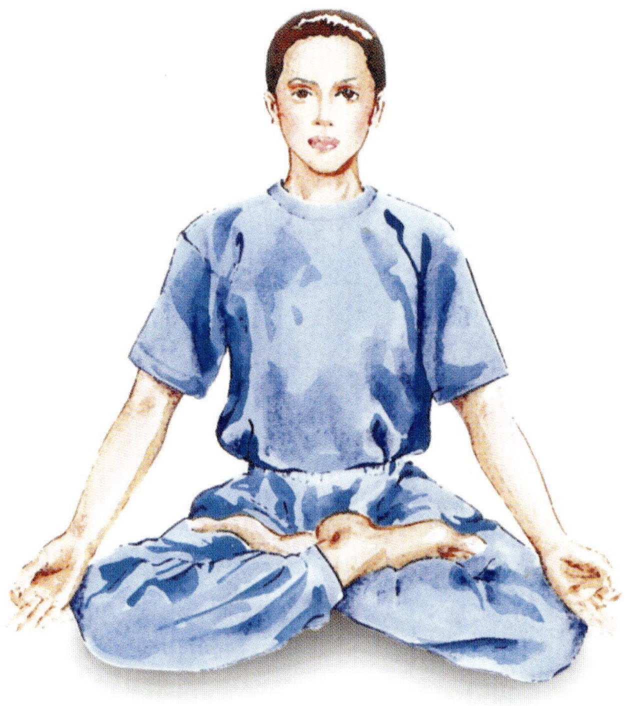

Padmasana: *Known popularly as the lotus pose or the meditation posture, this can be done by all. The subject should sit cross-legged on the floor, with each foot on the opposite thigh and heels as close to the groin as possible. The knees should touch the ground; facing upward, the palms must be placed on the knees, with the thumbs and index fingers held together in a circle.*

Paschimottanasana: *This is a back stretching posture. With legs stretched out in front while sitting, the subject raises both arms above the head, taking a deep breath. Exhaling, he/she bends forward, grasping the toes (or ankles), while making the forehead touch the knees.*

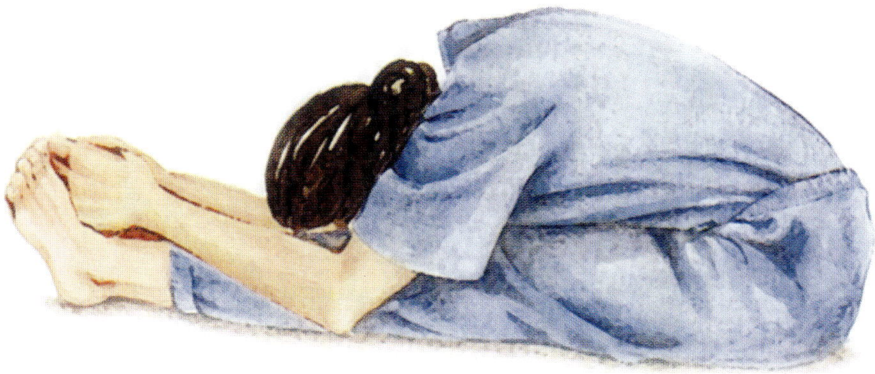

Shavasana: *The 'corpse pose' is a total relaxation method for the body and mind. Lying on the back, legs outstretched, heels together and toes a little apart, the arms should be placed alongside the body, palms facing upwards with the fingers limp and slightly curved. Eyes closed, the body should be allowed to relax in this position for 15 to 20 minutes.*

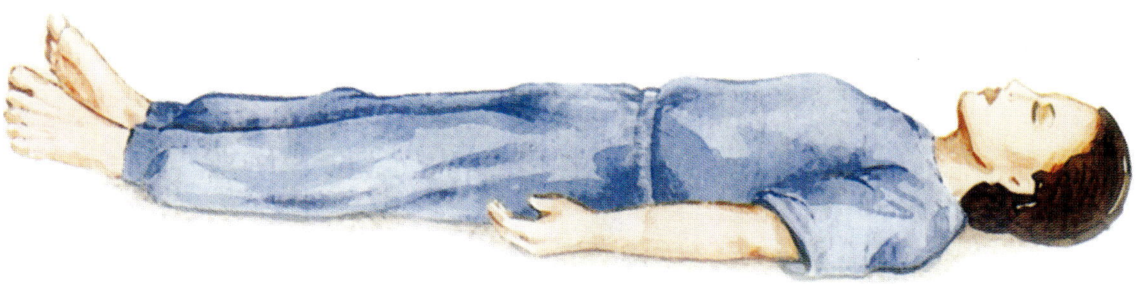

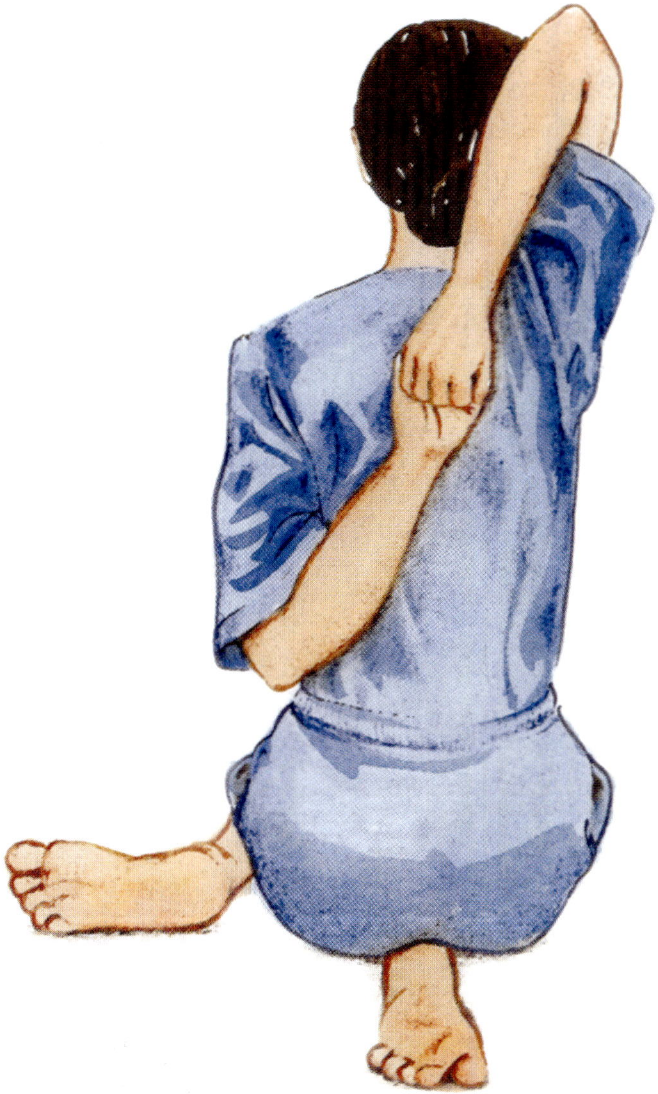

Gomukhasana: *Known as the cow-face posture (*gou *means cow and* mukha *means face in Sanskrit), this asana expands the lungs and is helpful in cases of asthma, high blood pressure and mental strain.*

Sitting on the floor, the subject should bend forward and raise the body, so that the weight rests on the hands. Passing the right flexed knee over the left one, the subject should then sit on the left heel, resting the body's weight on it. The soles must face upwards. Bending the right arm, the elbow should be held high and stretched over the right shoulder as far down the middle of the back as possible, keeping the spine straight. The left hand should then be brought up the centre of the back from below so that the hands meet, the palm of the right hand facing the back and the palm of the left hand facing outwards. The subject must keep looking in front.

Vshtrasana: *This is a spinal stretch. Lying on the stomach with the chin resting on the floor, the subject should flex the legs while gripping the ankle joints. The next step involves lifting the trunk and the legs as shown in the picture.*

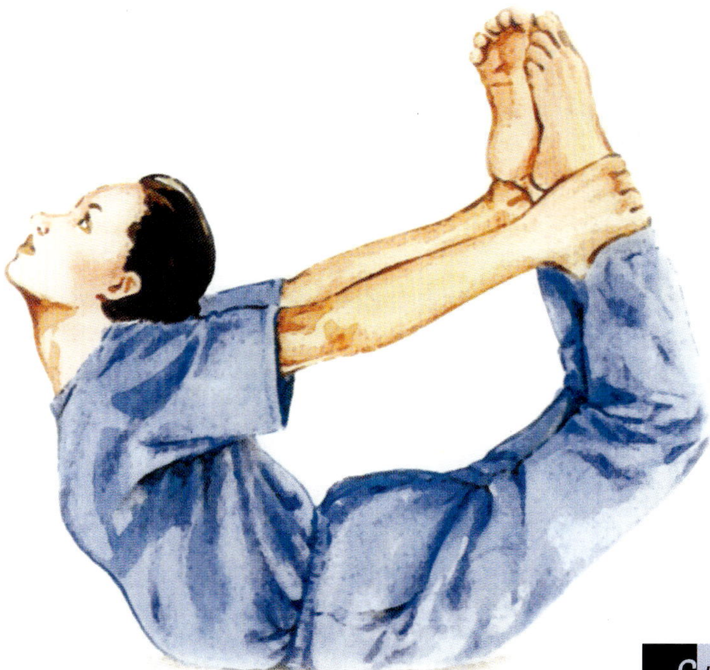

Some of the important *asanas* practised in our country are *Padmasana, Shavasana, Vshtrasana* and *Paschimottanasana.*

Padmasana and *Siddhasana* are used during meditation and *Pranayama* (breathing exercise), while *Shavasana* is the posture for achieving relaxation after doing the other *asanas*. It is also done at the end of the day.

Normally, *Shavasana* is recommended for 15-20 minutes, but even if you try it for 5-10 minutes, specially in the evening after a hard day's work, you will experience more physical and mental relaxation than you would with tranquillisers.

Shavasana for 5 to 10 minutes after a hard day's work relaxes you physically and mentally.

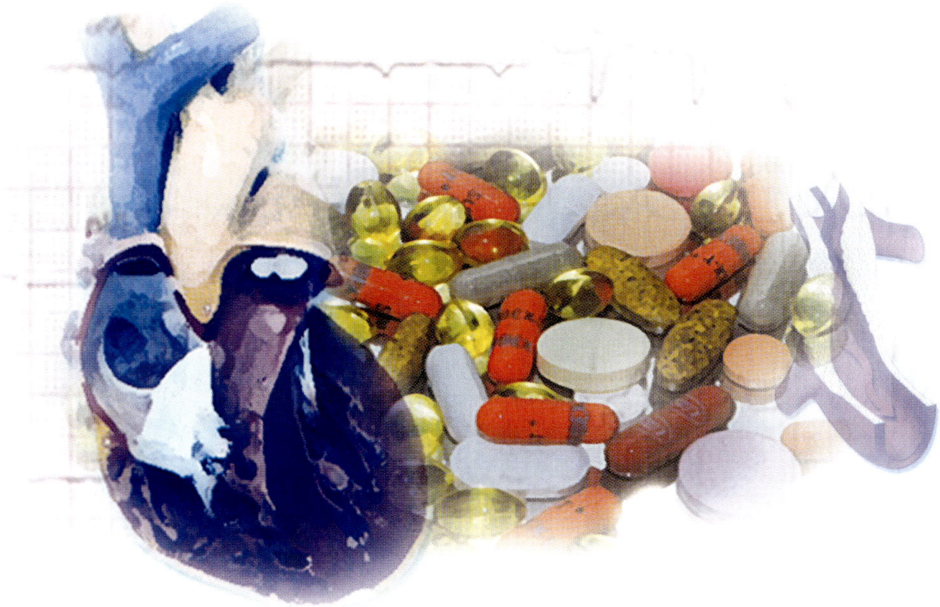

3. Common Heart Diseases

Heart disease is probably the most common cause of death today. Periodic check-ups can help a person to identify and check heart disease with the appropriate drug therapy or surgical intervention. For descriptive purposes heart diseases may be classified as:

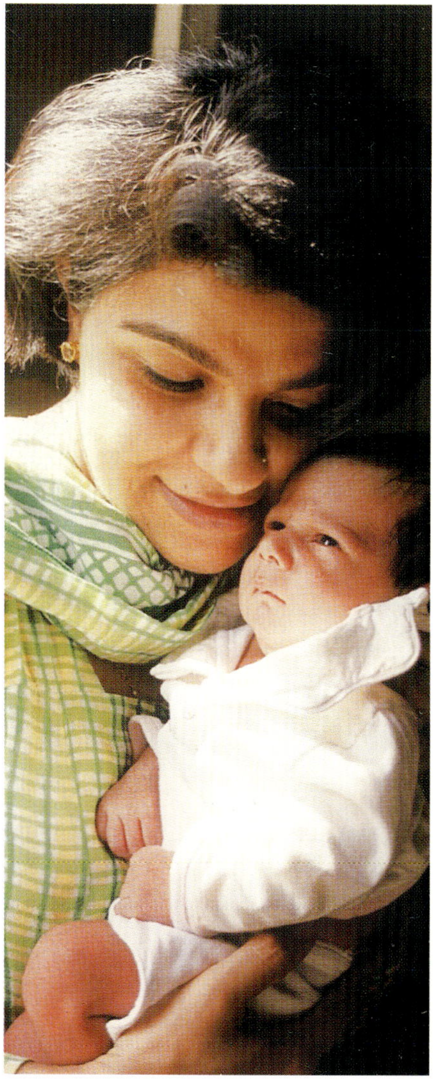

CONGENITAL HEART DISEASE

Those heart defects which are present at birth — that is, those which occur during the early development of the foetus during pregnancy — are called Congenital Heart Diseases. These defects include a hole in the heart, narrowed heart valves, malposition of a heart chamber or blood vessels and being born a blue baby. Such defects lead to a mixture of impure blood (venous) with pure (oxygenated) blood. Most of these cardiac defects are surgically correctable and some can be managed by non-surgical interventions like ballooning and other devices.

In fact many such heart diseases can be prevented by:

1. Avoiding the following during pregnancy:

- Alcohol
- Lithium (commonly used in depressive disorders)
- Amphetamines (synthetic drugs used as stimulants)
- Anti-convulsants
- Newer sedatives, tranquillisers or any other new drugs with unknown long-term effects on the foetus

2. Prevention and control of maternal diseases such as:

- Rubella (German measles)
- Diabetes

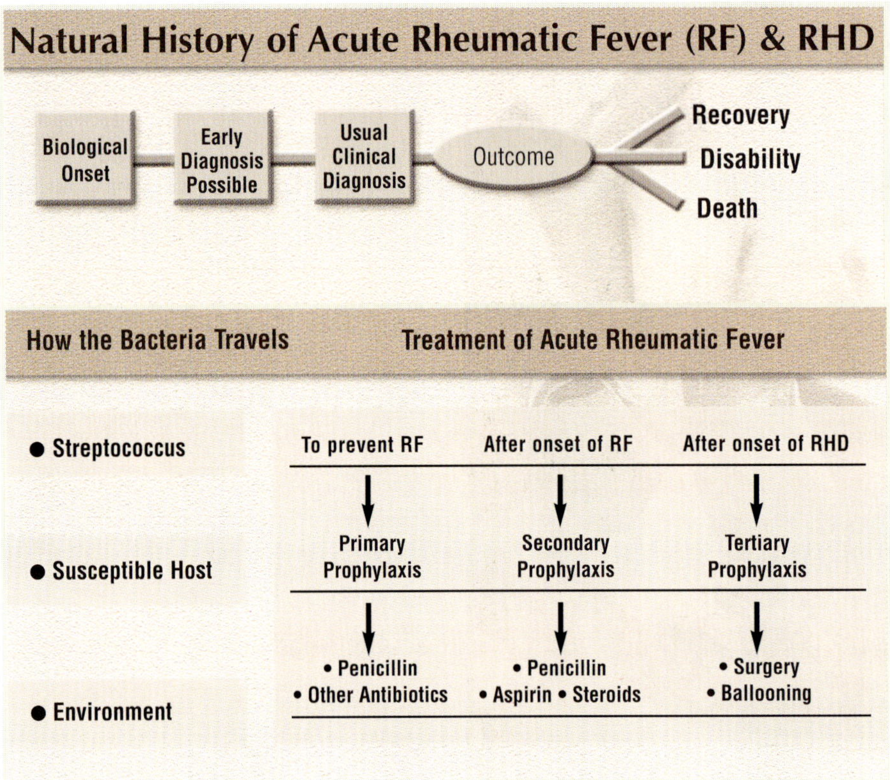

3. Genetic counselling in cases of:

- Parents having congenital heart defects
- Other siblings having such disorders

RHEUMATIC HEART DISEASE (RHD)

This is a disease of the heart valves or heart muscle due to rheumatic fever which is a result of sensitivity to bacterial sore throat infection during childhood and school-going age (5-15 years). It 'licks' the joints but 'bites' the heart. The joints only get temporarily swollen and painful but the heart valves bear the brunt of disease as they become either incompetent (leaky) or narrow. They can be corrected only through surgery or ballooning procedures.

CORONARY (ISCHAEMIC) HEART DISEASE OR ATHEROSCLEROSIS DISEASE

The heart muscle gets its nutrition through blood vessels called coronary arteries, of which there are mainly two: the right and left coronary arteries, but as the left, soon after its origin from the aorta, divides into two main branches called the Left Anterior Descending (LAD) and the Circumflex branch, conventionally they are described as three coronary arteries. Hence,

Treatment of Clogged Arteries

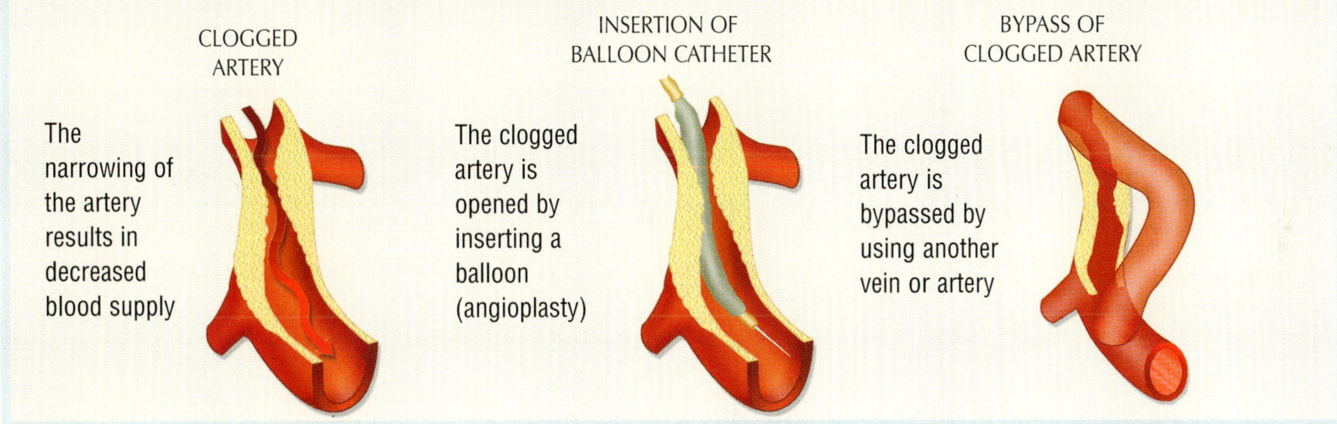

coronary artery disease can be a Single Vessel Disease (SVD), a Double Vessel Disease (DVD) or a Triple Vessel Disease (TVD). The narrowing of the coronary arteries due to the deposition of cholesterol and other blood fats, specially LDL (Low Density Lipoprotein), by a process called atherosclerosis is the major cause of heart attacks not only in industrialised countries but also in the developing world. This disease is also called ischaemic heart disease due to the fact that the process of atherosclerosis (narrowing) of arteries results in decreased blood supply (ischaemia). This leads to heart attacks (myocardial infarction), angina and heart failure.

Coronary heart disease includes conditions like heart attacks, angina pectoris, irregular heart beats and congestive heart failure.

Prevention of Coronary Heart Disease: Coronary artery disease and atherosclerosis can be prevented or reversed by:

- Avoiding smoking.
- Doing regular physical exercise and avoiding sedentary living habits.
- Taking a diet rich in vegetable fibre; complex carbohydrates like tubers and roots; and avoiding refined sugars, sucrose and fatty foods, excess of dairy products and red organ meat. This diet plan will check a rise in serum cholesterol which should be controlled

Non-Cardiac Causes of Chest Pain

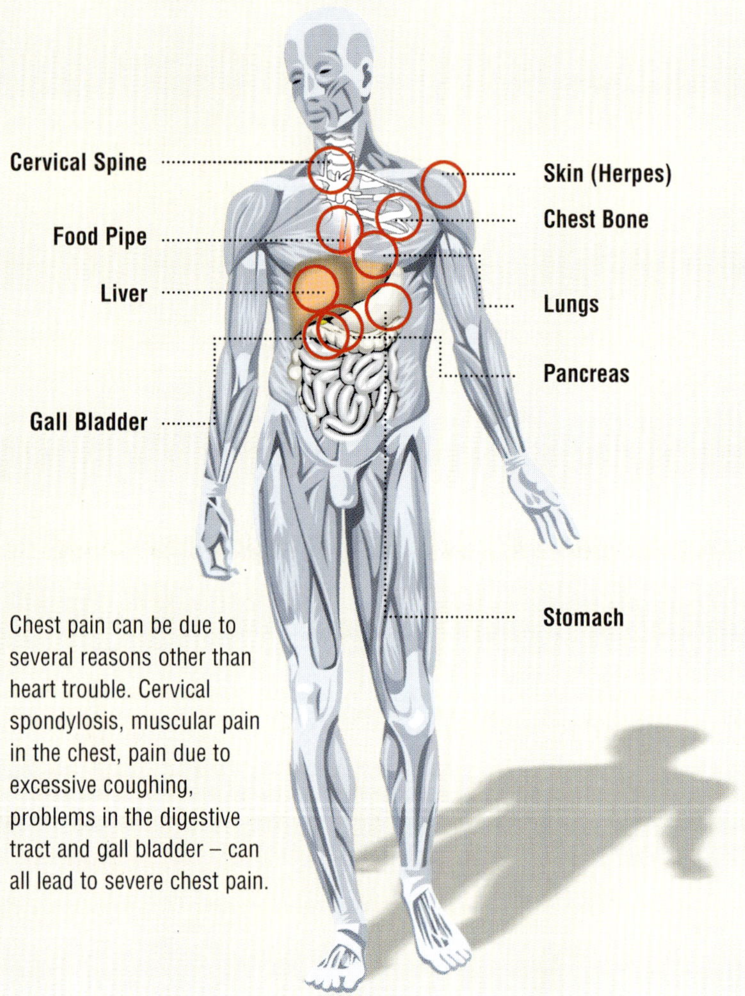

Chest pain can be due to several reasons other than heart trouble. Cervical spondylosis, muscular pain in the chest, pain due to excessive coughing, problems in the digestive tract and gall bladder – can all lead to severe chest pain.

preferably without drug therapy (see pages on diet).

- Early detection and effective control of diabetes, high blood pressure and gout, once again preferably by hygienic, non-drug measures.
- Practice of mental relaxation through yoga, music and meditation.
- Recurrence of heart attack can also be prevented (secondary prevention) by practice of the primary preventive measures as described above.

HYPERTENSION (HIGH BLOOD PRESSURE)

Normally the blood flows in the arteries under a certain pressure which in adults is less than 140/90 mm Hg. Repeated blood pressure readings of 140/90 mm Hg or above in an adult show that the individual is suffering from hypertension. High blood pressure left untreated results in increased chances of death and disability from stroke, heart attack and renal failure. There is no such entity as 'low blood pressure'; in fact if the blood pressure does not increase with age after adulthood, it is a healthy sign. If the blood pressure is suddenly found much lower than the usual normal for that person, one must rule out silent heart attack (see Chapter 4 on High Blood Pressure: The Silent Disease).

OTHER HEART PROBLEMS

Apart from the above, there are other heart problems such as **pericarditis**, a disease of the pericardium (the fibrous covering all around the heart), the major cause being tuberculosis. **Aortoarteritis**, the patchy narrowing of the arteries, the cause of which is unknown, results in secondary hypertension and ischaemia of the limbs, brain and abdominal organs, depending upon the culprit arteries. A **heart block** needing pacemaker treatment is yet another disease of the heart involving the nerve conduction system.

Cardiomyopathy (heart muscle disease) involves the contractile power of the heart muscle leading to its impairment, heart enlargement and decrease in the ejection power of blood. Often the only treatment for this disease is a heart transplant.

THE CARDINAL SYMPTOMS OF HEART DISEASE

The main symptoms indicating an underlying heart ailment are:

- Palpitations (uncomfortable awareness of the heartbeats)
- Breathlessness either during exertion or even at rest
- Chest pain
- Onset of undue fatigue in an otherwise apparently 'normal' person
- Blackouts or transient attacks of loss of consciousness (syncope).

Presence of any one or more of these symptoms should make one suspect heart disease and seek medical advice. It is worth mentioning here that any one or all these symptoms can occur in other diseases also in cases where there is an absolutely normal heart. So the mere occurrence of these symptoms should not create panic as they may occur due to anaemia (haemoglobin deficiency due to blood loss from any cause or due to impaired red blood cell formation), thyroid disease, lung diseases or mere anxiety states.

The genesis of these symptoms is the fact that the heart has to work under high pressure. This is more common in patients with hypertension or in cases of heart valve deformities, where an

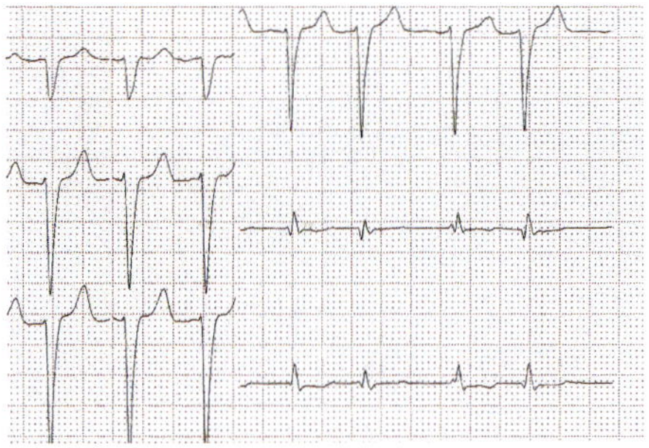

Electrocardiogram (ECG) *records the electrical activity of the heart as it contracts and rests.*

obstruction is created to the blood flow from or towards the heart such as in rheumatic and congenital heart disease. Symptoms of heart disease also arise when there is impaired nutrition of the heart muscle as happens in patients with narrowed coronary arteries (angina and heart attacks).

DIAGNOSIS OF HEART DISEASE

Missing the correct diagnosis of heart disease may prove disastrous. Incorrect diagnosis of heart disease when it does not exist is equally dangerous for the individual and for the family as this may cause a great deal of psychological trauma apart from unnecessary and expensive diagnostic testing and often, costly medication.

A doctor's examination: The most important aspect of a correct diagnostic approach is a carefully taken history and listening to the patient's story with a great deal of patience.

A physical examination: Next is the detailed physical examination from the toes to the head — toes first because feeling for the pulsations in the feet and legs provides vital information of the state of the arteries. Some cases of curable hypertension can be correctly diagnosed simply by feeling the peripheral pulsations and taking blood pressure in the legs in addition to the conventionally taken pressure in the arm. With the head, on the other extreme, looking into the eyes with an opthalmoscope

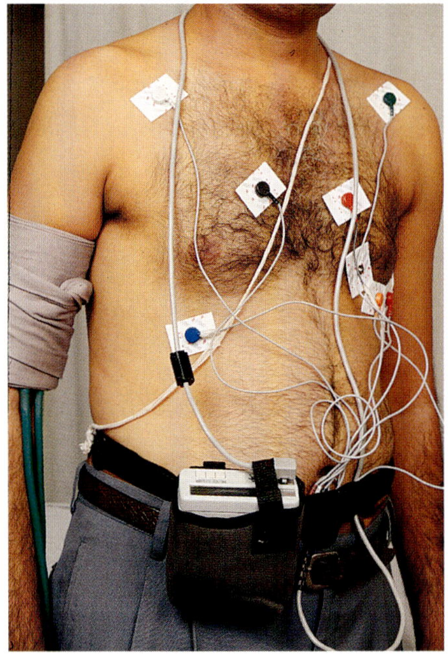

Holter Study *monitors the electrical activity of the heart for 24 hours.*

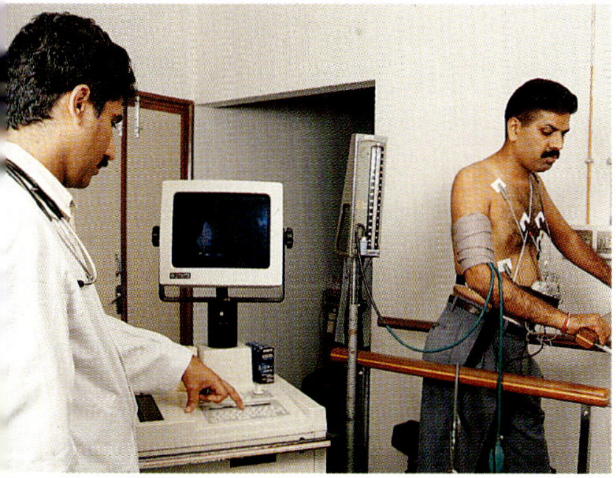

Tread Mill Test (TMT) *involves keeping a record of a person's speed while walking and increasing the speed to assess the workload he is capable of taking.*

reveals the severity of hypertension and certain complications of other heart diseases. By and large a reasonably correct diagnosis of heart disease can be made with a detailed history-taking and thorough physical examination. The various tests that help in confirming the diagnosis and ascertaining the severity of heart disease are as follows:

- ***Investigative blood tests:*** These will include a haemogram to see if the patient is anaemic as anaemia could be the cause of his symptoms and not heart disease, thyroid tests (T3, T4, TSH), blood sugar levels (for diabetes) and blood lipid profile (to check the cholesterol, triglycerides, lipoproteins), urea, uric acid, electrolytes (Na + Kt), as these are major coronary risk factors.
- ***ECG (Electrocardiogram):*** A normal resting ECG does not rule out a serious underlying heart disease.
- ***Holter Study:*** A 24-hour ambulatory ECG is a test in which the ECG is recorded continuously at work or at rest, during playing a game or during recreational activity. It is thus a very useful test in those patients who have symptoms of palpitation or chest pain at odd times during their work or during any tense situations where it is not

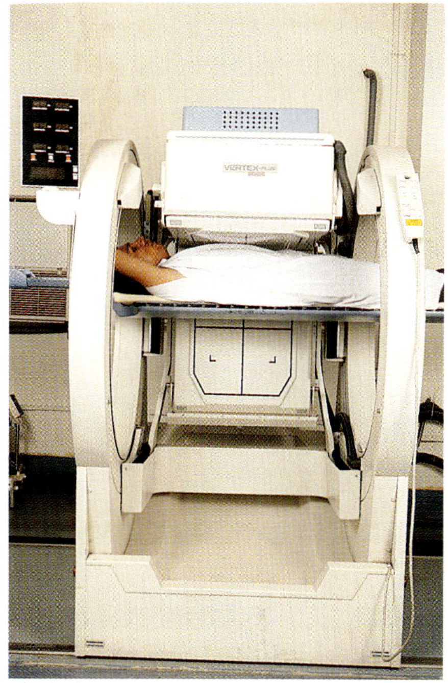

Echo Test *takes X-ray-like pictures which are obtained through sound waves. It reveals the pumping action of the heart and state of the heart valves.*

possible to use an ECG at that time. In this test a tape recorder is strapped to the patient and an event-marking diary is given to him. As his heart activities are being continously recorded, the patient makes a record of any symptoms he experiences during the next 24 or 36 hours depending upon the duration of tape (which is generally of 24 hours). An analysis of this record can tell us if the patient is experiencing any episode of reduced blood supply to his heart or any irregularity in his heart rhythm. Based on this ECG record the physician is able to advise the correct line of treatment. The Holter Study is also useful for follow-up of heart patients and to monitor the efficacy of drug treatment regimens.

- ***Tread Mill Test (TMT):*** A person with chest pain and normal ECG is advised this test which is helpful in making the correct diagnosis of any underlying heart disease.

- ***Stress Thallium Test:*** In some patients with chest discomfort but a normal ECG at rest and a negative Tread Mill Test (TMT) report, or when the TMT cannot be done due to certain reasons, a radio isotope test named Stress Thallium Test is done. Either thallium is injected during peak exercise time or medicines are given that push up the heart rate and blood pressure, simulating what happens during exercise. Through the Stress Thallium Test one can find out whether the blood supply to various parts of the heart is normal or impaired. This indicates the absence or presence of any blocks in the major blood vessels supplying the heart muscle, thus helping us to plan future management strategies.

- ***Fluoroscopy and Ultra Fast CT Scan:*** This screening test is useful for diagnosing coronary disease by detecting calcification in the coronary arteries.

- ***Cardiac Catheterisation and Coronary Angiography:*** A patient with chest pain or chest discomfort on exertion or at rest, and with an abnormal TMT, must undergo the test of coronary angiography which indicates the exact site and extent of blocks in the coronary arteries. This test is done by introducing a small tube (catheter) through the groin / arm artery into the coronary arteries and injecting a radio-opaque material through it into the coronary artery and taking a run with a cine film or on a CD. This is then viewed through a projector and an impression made of the site and extent of blocks in the coronary arteries. The state of the heart muscle can also be gauged by doing a left ventricular angiogram by the same procedure. Sometimes a coronary angiography may be advised even if the TMT and thallium tests are negative but the patient is still suffering from a very annoying type of chest pain.

AREAS OF PAIN

Most often the pain is felt in the centre of the chest, behind the breastbone. Sometimes it travels along both the shoulders to the inner side of the arms right up to the fingers. The pain is felt more acutely in the left arm than the right arm, the neck and in the back in-between the shoulder blades. Occasionally this pain may be felt in the jaw, the molar teeth or in the upper part of the abdomen.

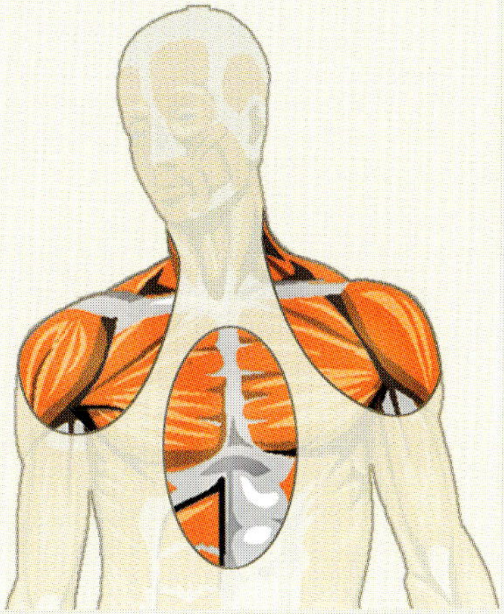

■ ***Angiography of other arteries:*** This is carried out specially in the aorta and renal (kidney) arteries in some cases of hypertension to detect any curable cause of high blood pressure and to plan treatment accordingly.

■ ***CT Scan of abdominal organs:*** This is advised in some cases of hypertension to detect any tumours or narrowing of renal arteries, both conditions being amenable to curable treatment.

A person with symptoms of chest pain, palpitation, breathlessness or undue fatigue should not neglect these early warnings of underlying heart disease. The advised investigations must be done so that the correct diagnosis of heart disease can be arrived at during the early stages and proper treatment advised accordingly so as to prevent any serious eventualities.

TREATMENT OF HEART DISORDERS

Angina

Angina or *angina pectoris* are words which come from the Greek *angiousus* meaning strangulation or suffocation and *pectoris* meaning chest. The term, therefore, refers to suffocation, hunger for air or a strangulation-like feeling in the chest. The angina pain usually comes on with exertion and subsides on resting. The chest discomfort or pain of acute heart attack (myocardial infarction) on the other hand, mostly occurs at rest, generally lasting for more than half an hour compared to anginal pain which lasts only for a few minutes, subsiding soon after rest or putting a tablet of nitroglycerine below the tongue.

Areas of Pain: Most often the pain is felt in the centre of the chest,

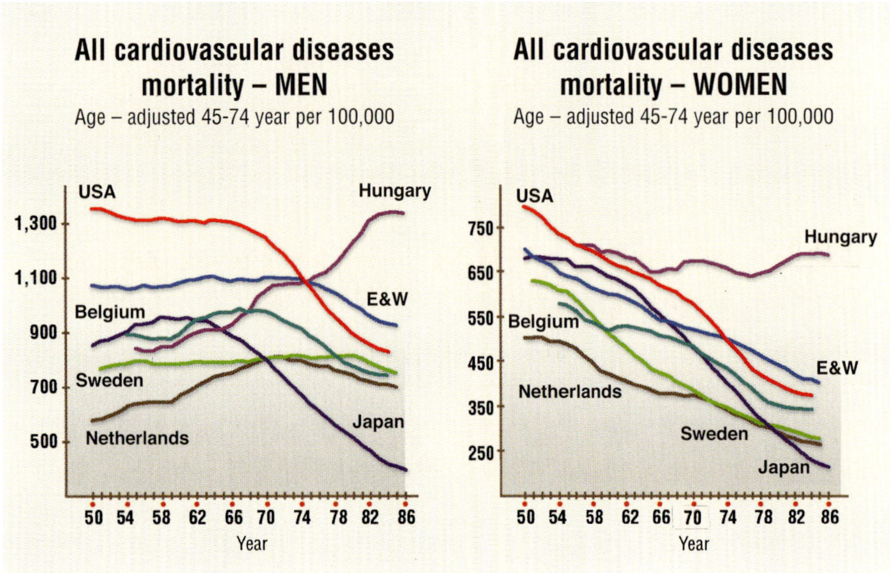

behind the breastbone. Sometimes it travels along both the shoulders to the inner side of the arms right up to the fingers. The pain is felt more acutely in the left arm than the right arm. In fact the pain may also radiate to the neck and in the back in-between the shoulder blades. Occasionally this pain may be felt in the jaw, the molar teeth or in the upper part of the abdomen.

It is important to understand that every chest pain is not angina as conditions like cervical spondylosis, muscular pain, gall bladder disease, stomach ulcer and diseases like pleurisy or other inflammations within the chest or in the structures like the skin, bone, muscles, nerves and lungs near or adjacent to the heart may result in chest pain akin to chest disease. A carefully listened-to history of the patient will help in making the correct diagnosis of *angina pectoris* and acute heart attack. The classical description of an anginal attack is the pain or chest discomfort like a suffocating feeling in a wider region of the chest, either in the centre or left side, or the jaws or arms, left side more than the right and not as a pin-pointed localised pain. The pain comes on either due to physical effort or mental tension, subsiding with rest or taking a nitrate tablet. If this chest discomfort does not subside with rest or one or two tablets of nitrates (one should not take more than two at a time as that may result in fall in blood pressure), or the pain which starts while resting and continues for over 15 minutes, one should suspect it to be a case of acute myocardial infarction (heart attack). The patient should be given a tablet of aspirin to chew (if he is not suffering from a stomach ulcer) and immediately shown to a doctor or moved into a hospital equipped with facilities to treat patients with acute heart attacks.

It is important to realise that the treatment for acute heart attack must start at the earliest without any delay as a delay of even a few minutes can adversely affect the outcome in recovery and may result in irreversible damage to the heart muscle.

Apart from drugs like nitrates, beta blockers, calcium channel blockers, ace inhibitors, anti-platelet agents and nitric oxide liberators, intervention procedures and devices like angioplasty (ballooning), use of stents, laser radiation therapy with beta and gamma rays, bypass surgery and transmyocardial revascularisation (increasing blood supply to the heart muscle) have established a definite role in the modern management of patients with angina, giving them not only a better quality of life but also a longer life.

TREATMENT OF HEART ATTACK (ACUTE MYOCARDIAL INFARCTION)

It is extremely important not to confuse a heart attack with gas or muscular pain as this may be disastrous. A patient complaining of severe chest discomfort, not necessarily pain, acute suffocation or a feeling of heavy weight in the chest should be given a nitrate tablet. The same applies to anyone who experiences severe chest pain which may radiate to the jaws and arms, more on the left side than the right or back, while resting or even during exertion and lasting for mostly over half an hour. If the patient does not improve with the nitrate tablet and rest, he must be suspected of suffering from an acute heart attack and should be given immediate medical relief. He should preferably be moved to the nearest medical centre equipped for patients with heart attacks as much more than just morphine, oxygen and bedrest would be required.

Present-day management of a patient with acute heart attack (myocardial infarction) broadly comprises:

Administration of thrombolytic agents (clot busters): The most common cause of acute heart attack is clogging of a coronary artery with a fresh thrombus (clot) over an already underlying atherosclerotic plaque. These drugs fall under the category of clot busters (streptokinase and urokinase) and their rapidly changing new versions with more clot-specific actions.

Primary angioplasty (ballooning): This can be done with or without intracoronary stents. An open blood vessel is any day better than a partly open or a blocked vessel. With thrombolytic (clot buster) therapy one is not certain of opening the vessel in all cases. The surer way these days is the opening of the freshly blocked (occluded) vessel with a balloon (angioplasty) and placing a coil-like element (stent) in the opened artery so that it does not close down again. When this procedure is done within about six or preferably four hours after the onset of chest discomfort of a heart attack, we can prevent damage to the heart muscle, thus rendering it totally unaffected in spite of the fact that the person has suffered a heart attack. This is possible to achieve by early intervention in restoring the normal blood supply to the heart muscle by procedures such as primary angioplasty.

Surgery: Since the introduction of ballooning angioplasty the role of cardiac surgery in the treatment of acute myocardial infarction has become minimal, except in situations when a heart attack gets complicated with heart valve or heart muscle ruptures and where surgical operative procedures prove life saving.

Medicines: Used in the treatment of acute heart attack, they include analgesics and sedatives like morphine or pethidine, oxygen, anti-clotting agents like aspirin and heparin. There are drugs that help in improving the heart muscle functioning after a heart attack by varied mechanism; others are useful in preventing another heart attack (secondary prevention), including beta blockers, ace inhibitors, some calcium channel blockers, potassium channel openers, nitrates and other nitric oxide liberators.

Lipid-lowering drugs: Three types of lipoproteins (fats combined with proteins) carry cholesterol from the liver to different parts of the body through the blood. Low Density Lipoprotein (LDL) is the most cholesterol-rich lipoprotein and slowly gets deposited in the walls of the arteries, resulting in their

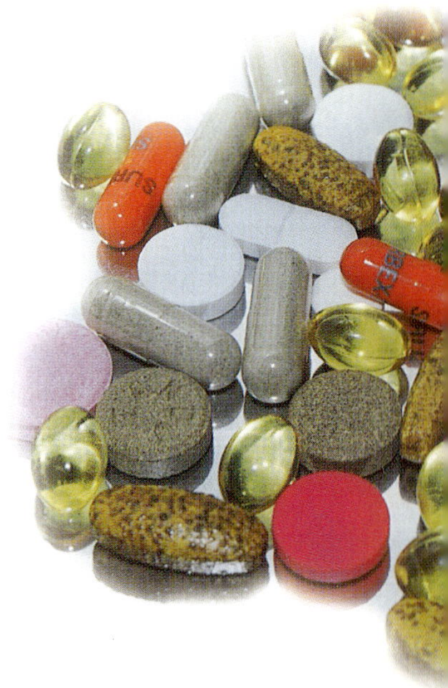

clogging. It is popularly, therefore, known as 'bad' cholesterol. High Density Lipoprotein (HDL) or 'good' cholesterol, is formed in the liver. It obtains cholesterol from the surrounding tissue, is then transported through the blood back to the liver, from where cholesterol is excreted in the bile.

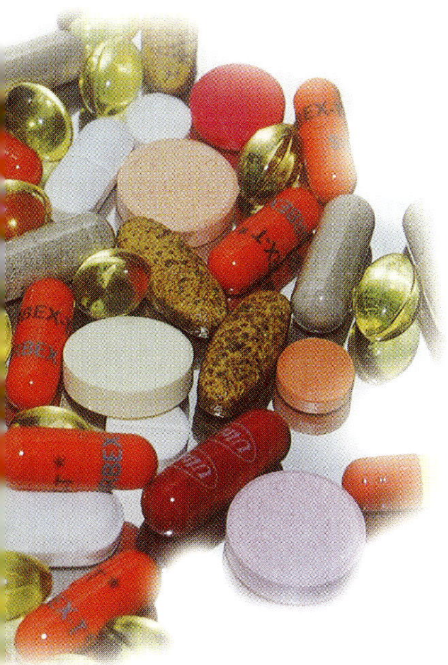

Triglycerides are a type of fat produced by the liver. The famous Framingham Study found that a high triglyceride level was a significant risk for coronary heart disease. High blood cholesterol and high levels of LDL (Low Density Lipoprotein) and low HDL (High Density Lipoprotein) have been found to be closely related to the occurrence of heart attacks through the process of atherosclerosis. Drugs that lower the LDL and total cholesterol and increase HDL levels in blood have been reported to both prevent the first occurrence of heart attacks (primary prevention) as well as to prevent the recurrence when being used after the first heart attack (secondary prevention). Notable among these drugs are: Nicotinic acid, Gemfibrozil, Bizafibrozil and Statins. It is the use of Statins, Lovaslatin, Simvostation, Pravastion and Atorvastatin — specially Atorvastatin — that has resulted in lesser number of patients going for angioplasty after they started using this medicine. Long-term use of such cholesterol-lowering drugs should be closely monitored with periodic blood tests for any liver or muscle damage.

Supportive measures: Along with the drugs mentioned above, supportive measures such as (i) regular physical exercise; (ii) diet control to avoid overeating, excess salt, alcohol, sugar and fatty foods; (iii) avoiding smoking and (iv) mental relaxation through meditation, music, attending religious congregations and practice of yoga, are common to the management of patients with angina and acute heart attack and also for primary prevention of these diseases.

TREATMENT OF OTHER HEART DISEASES

Excellent intervention procedures and devices are available for the treatment of practically all heart diseases. The various means available are:

1. Ballooning valvotomy for narrowed heart valves due to congenital cardiac defects or as a result of rheumatic heart disease.

2. Umbrella and other types of devices like coils to plug the various defects or holes inside the heart and blood vessels.

3. Coils to strengthen the weak portion of blood vessels to prevent their expansion or bursting, leading to severe and often fatal bleeding.

4. Pacemakers are used to increase the heart rates to desirable levels in those patients who have blackouts or become unconscious due to sudden fall in their pulse rates.

5. Some heart patients suffer from attacks of sudden rise in their pulse rate and irregular and rapid heartbeats. In the past they used to be treated throughout their lives with drug therapy which often had side-effects on other organs and even on the heart. These days such patients can be permanently cured by the use of techniques called Radio Frequency Ablation (RFA) and in such cases they do not require any drug therapy.

6. Some heart patients may suddenly die due to a serious heart rhythm problem called ventricular techycardia leading to ventricular fibrillation or a fast, chaotic, practically ineffective contraction of the heart which is a sure cause of sudden death. At present there are devices called automatic implantable cardioverter-defibrillators which when given to a patient, can detect and abolish this serious heart disorder, thus averting sudden death.

All these devices have revolutionised the management of patients with heart ailments giving them a better quality of life and prolonging their life.

7. There are powerful drugs available for treatment of heart failure and lately the introduction of ace inhibitors and spironolactone have dramatically changed the situation of patients suffering from heart failure. With the use of these drugs some patients who were candidates for a heart transplant did not in fact need it.

8. Heart Transplant: For end-stage heart failure patients where medicines do not help, there is the final hope of treatment with a cardiac transplant. As the availability of a donor heart is always a big problem and unpredictable, in future its place will be taken by a mechanical heart. This is already being used in some patients.

Gene therapy is also on its way to help such patients.

THE THIRD DIMENSION: DOCTOR'S DEDICATION

Mere availability of drugs and devices does not suffice for optimum heart care. Nothing can replace the devotion of the physician handling the devices and other therapeutic interventions and his ability to reassure the patient and his family that the patient is getting the best available treatment.

EARLY DETECTION OF HEART DISEASE

1. Patients must describe at length and in detail their symptoms to their physicians. The chief symptoms for heart disease are palpitation, chest pain, breathlessness and undue fatigue.

2. Physicians must get into the habit of listening with patience to their patient's problems and doing a detailed physical examination to detect the underlying cause of the symptoms. Apart from coronary heart disease there are other cardiac and non-cardiac diseases (anaemia, thyroid problems and gross obesity) which would present the same symptoms of palpitation, breathlessness, fatigue and chest pain like in cases of heart attacks.

Treatment for acute heart attack must start at the earliest: any delay may cause irreversible damage to the heart and even be fatal.

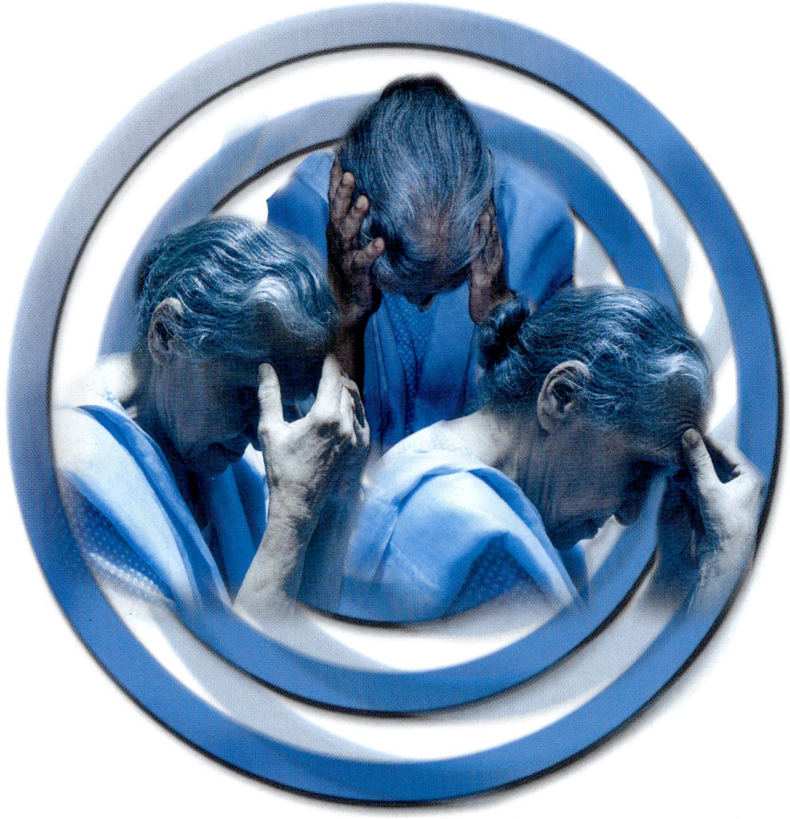

4. High Blood Pressure: The Silent Disease

Blood pressure is also known as hypertension. Under circumstances of a hostile environment, a stressful or annoying situation or provocative remarks, a person may feel restless, be unable to concentrate, have shaky hands, a red face and flushed eyes and feel heaviness in the head or develop a pulsatile headache. These symptoms are usually the manifestation of a state when the blood circulation in the body is at a pressure higher than what that individual is normally used to in day-to-day life. That brings us to the question: What is normal blood pressure? An approximate guide for adults used to be 100+age for the upper (systolic) pressure. Most world authorities including the World Health Organisation (WHO) now agree that in adults normal blood pressure is less than 140/90 mm Hg. If repeated blood pressure readings (at least three) on different occasions are found to be 140/90 mm Hg or above, the individual is said to be suffering from high blood pressure or hypertension. Several studies as well as Life Insurance statistics have shown that as the pressure goes on rising above this figure, life expectancy starts falling with increased morbidity and mortality due to high blood pressure mainly from stroke, heart failure and kidney disease. It is also true, however, that if blood pressure is adequately controlled with drugs or other means and kept below 140/90 mm Hg, many lives can be saved from death and disability due to stroke, heart and kidney failure.

Symptoms

High blood pressure is generally a 'silent disease', specially when it develops over a long time. Sometimes it is detected during a routine check-up. At other times if a person is suffering from **headaches, heaviness in the head, impairment in vision, disturbed sleep or lack of it, loss of concentration in work, heavy breathing during work or climbing stairs,** the physician should take the blood pressure readings with caution and care. If a person has one or more of these symptoms and one blood pressure reading is normal, the doctor must take more frequent readings to ascertain that at least three readings at three different times remain below 140/90 mm Hg before declaring that the individual has normal blood pressure. The reverse is more important: if the first blood pressure reading taken in the doctor's office or in the hospital is high, one must get it rechecked preferrably in homely surroundings and a friendly atmosphere and if these readings are normal, this may be just a case of 'White Coat Hypertension'—where fear, anxiety, apprehension and tension often tend to raise the blood pressure. Both the patient and the doctor should be in a relaxed and comfortable position during blood pressure measurement.

Causes of High Blood Pressure

Unlike diseases like typhoid, TB and malaria where we know the precise cause of the disease and the specific drug treatment, in the case of high blood pressure, no cause is known but we do have effective drugs and other means to treat this condition.

RISK FACTORS

- Overweight
- Sedentary lifestyle and lack of physical exercise
- Excessive alcohol consumption of more than two ounces of whisky/or other spirits in a day
- Excessive salt intake
- Repeated exposure to stressful situations at work or at home
- Cigarette smoking

When high blood pressure is found in children and young adults, there is generally a causative factor like some abnormality in the major blood vessels of the body or those of the kidneys, or a tumour in and around the kidneys. In such situations blood pressure can be permanently cured by ballooning methods or by surgery. In adults, however, such cases are rare. Certain risk factors, however, when present, make the person more prone to get high blood pressure.

Treatment

When a patient is diagnosed as having high blood pressure, the following investigations must be carried out which will help: (a) to find a possible cause for the high blood pressure and thereby focus in on a specific treatment in the form of ballooning (angioplasty) or

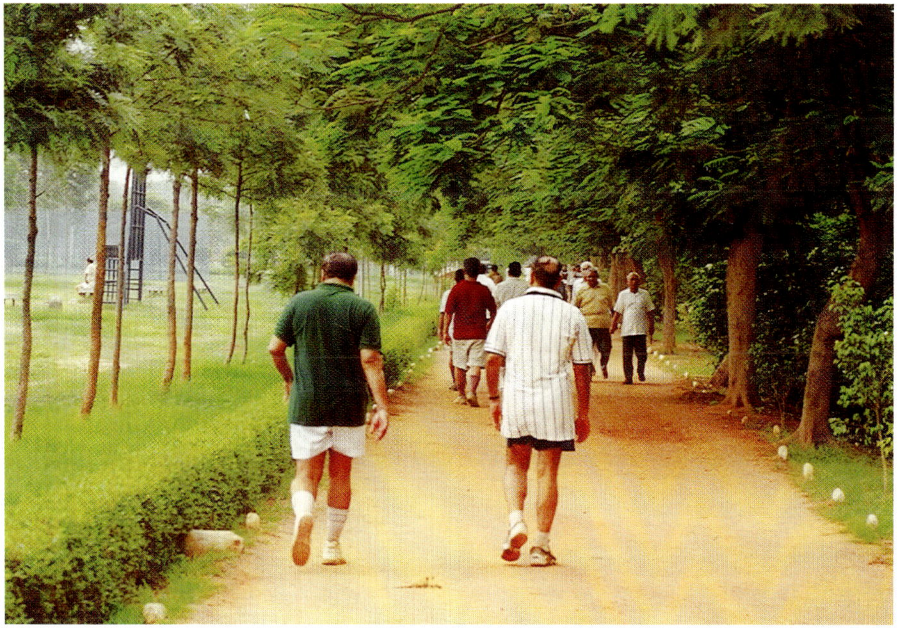

surgery and (b) to know the extent of damage done by high blood pressure to the vital organs such as the brain, eyes, heart and kidneys.

The investigations include:

1. Blood tests for haemogram, urea, sugar, uric acid, electrolytes (Na^+, K^+) and lipid profile—that is, cholesterol, triglycerides and lipoproteins like LDL, HDL and VLDL

2. Urine analysis for albumin and microscopy

3. X-rays of the chest and abdomen

4. ECG

5. Ultrasound of the abdomen to examine the kidneys and the adrenal glands

6. Eye check-up (Fundoscopy)

7. CT scan MRI and radioisotope renography when high blood pressure is suspected to be due to a tumour in the kidney or a vascular cause

Detailed investigations are an integral part of the treatment as they help the doctor to follow the correct line of treatment.

The actual treatment then comprises:

- Non-drug measures
- Drugs for high blood pressure
- Angioplasty with stents (ballooning)
- Surgery

The non-drug measures for treatment of high blood pressure include:

1. Weight reduction in those who are overweight

2. Doing regular physical exercise,

specially brisk walks, swimming and other dynamic exercises

3. Avoiding excess salt and alcohol

4. Practice of mental relaxation through meditation, music, yoga, study of religious scriptures and attending religious congregations

Drugs

Medical practitioners should prescribe only those drugs and drug combinations which do not cause any disturbances in blood glucose, cholesterol and electrolytes. One common side-effect of some blood pressure-lowering drugs is an adverse effect on the male erectile function. In case of this side-effect, other medicines from among the long list available should be given as a substitute.

When treating high blood pressure in elderly patients, the doctor must start with smaller doses of the drug and prescribe only one drug. The elderly cannot tolerate sudden fall in blood pressure and may develop adverse symptoms due to sudden decrease in blood supply to the brain if their blood pressure is brought down suddenly. The elderly are also more prone to hypotension, that is, sudden fall in blood pressure on standing. They should, therefore, be instructed to gradually adopt the standing posture from a supine position, preferably sitting in the bed with legs hanging down for a few seconds before standing up and walking.

STEP-DOWN THERAPY

Unlike the old concept that once blood pressure drugs are started, they will have to be continued for life, today it is possible to reduce the drug intake and, at times, even stop them while simultaneously continuing the recommended lifestyle modifications. Any reduction in or discontinuation of drug therapy should, however, be done only under medical supervision.

BALLOONING AND STENTING

Those patients whose high blood pressure is due to narrow or blocked arteries, specially the renal (kidney) arteries, can be successfully treated by angioplasty procedures, that is, ballooning and using metallic coils called stents to prevent recurrence of the narrowing. This procedure can be done at any age, including in the elderly, where the narrowing of the arteries is due to atherosclerosis.

Normal blood pressure in an adult should be below 140/90 mm Hg.

SURGERY

In rare cases high blood pressure is due to tumours in the kidneys or the neighbouring organs called adrenal glands; these cases can be cured of high blood pressure by operative procedures.

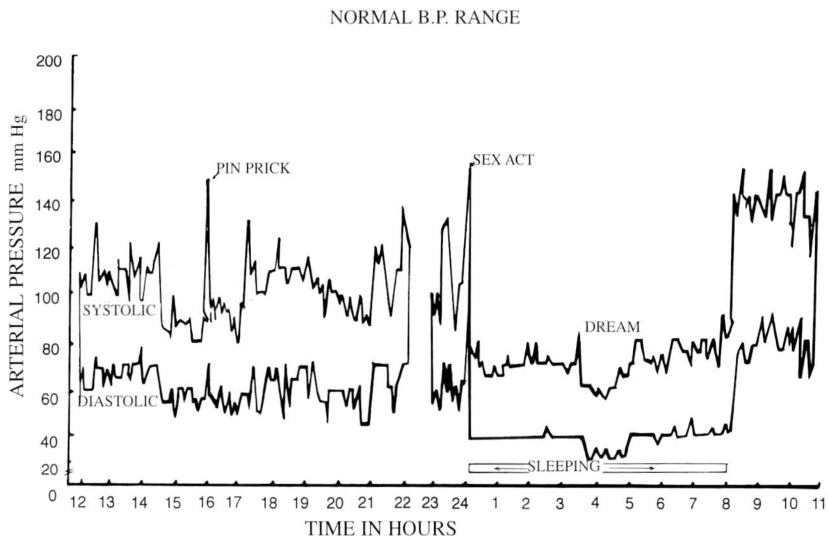

24 Hours Blood Pressure Record

LOW BLOOD PRESSURE

Medically there is no such disease called Low Blood Pressure. Normally blood pressure rises with age but in certain individuals it does not and that is probably due to a healthier lifestyle and habits. A blood pressure of 120/80 mm Hg in a healthy 80 year old is not a low blood pressure. However, when an individual with a normal blood pressure of 140/85 mm Hg, one day suddenly finds that his blood pressure has fallen to 110/70 mm Hg, this is definitely a fall in his blood pressure and must be investigated. The actual cause has to be discovered: is it due to severe dehydration, excessive sweating, fasting, internal or external bleeding or a silent heart attack?

Prevention of High Blood Pressure

The precise prevention of a disease can only be undertaken when the exact cause is known. Since the exact cause of high blood pressure is not known, the only preventive measures that can be taken are to guard against the risk factors (see p. 42) which either aggravate or initiate high blood pressure. A good indicator of your stress level is the following questionnaire:

ARE YOU UNDER STRESS?

Life's Stresses	Point Value of Stress
Death of spouse	**100**
Divorce	**73**
Marital separation from mate	**65**
Detention in jail or other institution	**63**
Death of a close family member	**63**
Major personal injury or illness	**53**
Marriage adjustments	**50**
Being fired at work	**47**
Marital reconciliation with mate	**45**
Retirement of work	**45**
Major change in health or behaviour of a family member	**44**
Foreclosure on a mortgage or loan	**30**
Pregnancy	**40**
Sexual difficulties	**39**
Gaining a new family member through birth, adoption, or older person moving in, etc.	**39**
Major personal readjustment — merger, reorganisation, bankruptcy, etc.	**39**
Death of a close friend	**32**
Changing to a different line of work	**36**
Major change in the number of arguments with spouse — a lot more or a lot less than usual	**35**
Vacation organisation	12
Taking on a large mortgage for purchasing a home, business, etc.	**31**
Major change in responsibilities at work — promotion, demotion, lateral transfer, etc.	**29**

Life's Stresses	Point Value of Stress
In-law troubles	**29**
Son or daughter leaving home — marriage, attending college, etc.	**29**
Outstanding personal achievement	**28**
Wife beginning or ceasing work outside home	**26**
Beginning or ceasing formal schooling	**26**
Major change in living conditions — building a home, repairs, deterioration of house or neighbourhood	**25**
Revision of personal habits, dress, manners, associations, etc.	**24**
Troubles with the boss	**23**
Major change in financial state — worse or better off than earlier	**38**
Major change in working hours or conditions	**20**
Change in residence	**20**
Changing to a new school	**20**

Life's Stresses	Point Value of Stress
Major change in type and amount of recreation	**19**
Major change in religious activities — a lot more or less than usual	**19**
Major change in social activities — clubs, dancing, movies, visiting, etc.	**18**
Taking on a large mortgage or loan for purchasing a car, TV, fridge, etc.	**17**
Major change in sleeping habits — a lot more or less sleep, or change in sleep timings	**16**
Major change in number of family get-togethers — a lot more or less than usual	**15**
Major change in eating habits — a lot more or less food intake; different meal hours or surroundings	**13**
Major festivals, e.g. Diwali, X'mas, etc.	**13**
Minor violation of the law — traffic tickets, jaywalking, disturbing the peace, etc.	**11**

Interpretation: Low stress: **0-140,** Mild stress: **150-199,** Moderate stress: **200-299,** Major stress: **300 or more**

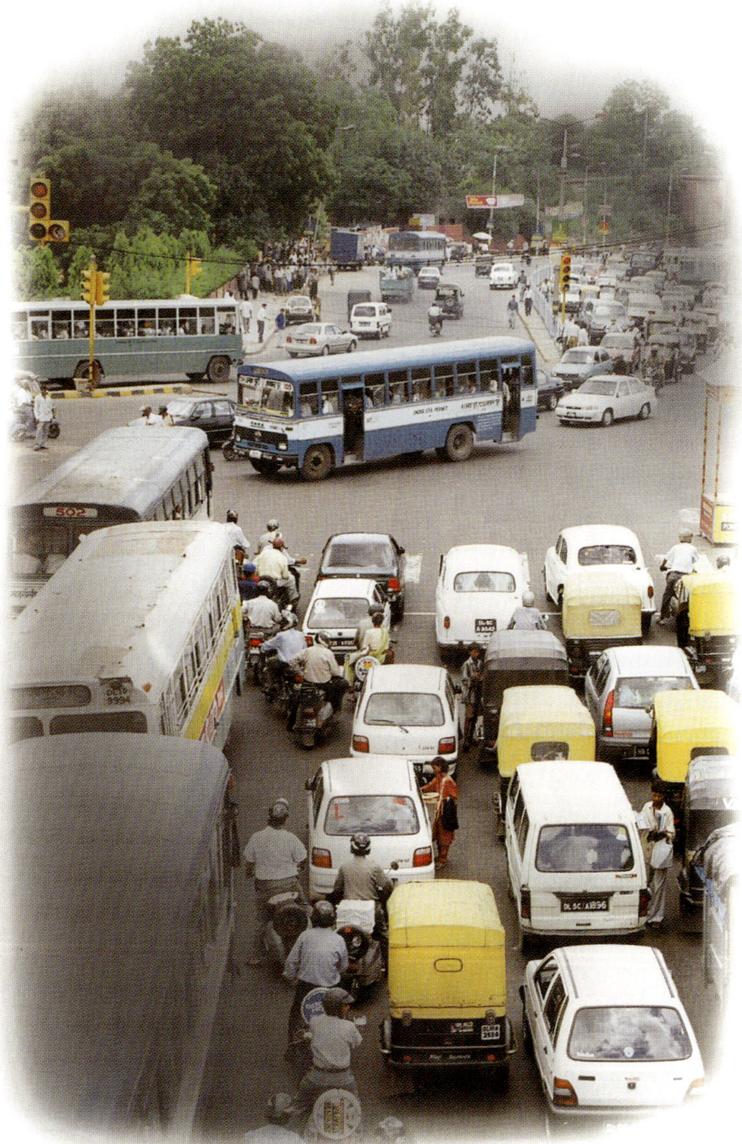
502

5. Environmental Pollution: The Heart's Enemy

Life thrives on two types of environment: the external environment from which the organism gets its food and air to survive, and the internal environment—the milieu interior which regulates the various metabolic processes at the cellular and mitochondrial level for life to be sustained. In broad terms, health is defined as the state of physical, mental and social well-being and not necessarily the absence of disease and infirmity (WHO). Sickness or disease, can be defined as: The structural and/or functional abnormality with the implication that the abnormality produced has the potential of lowering the quality of life contributing to a disabling illness or leading to death. Disturbances in the environment, including air pollution, affect health adversely in general and the heart in particular.

Heart Diseases and the Environment

A heart disease is not necessarily genetic; it is largely due to the effects of environmental factors, including: *Air pollution; Nutritional factors*—including over and under-nutrition; *Psychological behaviour factors* like hostility and negative emotions such as anger, greed, undue desires, attachment to materialistic things and maladjustment to daily challenges of life.

While psycho-social factors and living habits such as over-nutrition, smoking and sedentary lifestyles are more related to coronary heart diseases and hypertension, living in an overcrowded environment, coupled with poor nutrition, is responsible for a higher incidence of rheumatic fever and rheumatic heart disease which still has a high prevalence in India, while diseases of affluence like hypertension and coronary heart disease have also invaded us in an epidemic form. Control over environmental factors, including the food we eat, the water we drink and the air we breathe, go a long way in managing and preventing many cardiovascular disorders.

Hippocrates, the father of medicine (6th century B.C.), wisely stressed the role of the environment on health when he stated, 'Whoever wishes to study medicine well, should proceed thus: In the first place to consider the Seasons of the year . . . The Waters . . . The Ground and the Mode in which the

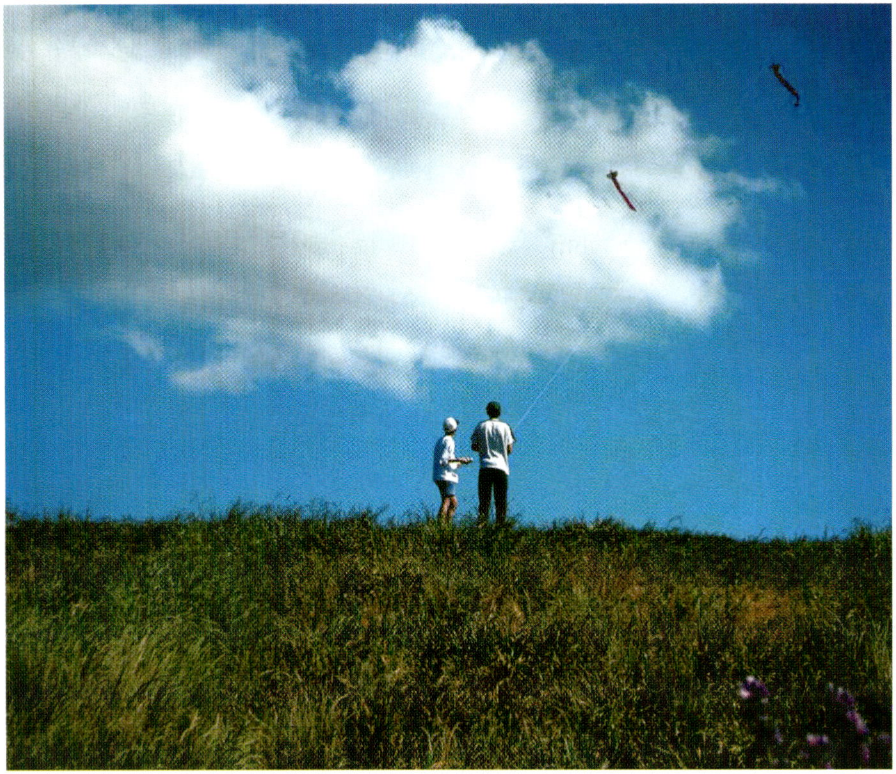

inhabitants live and what are their pursuits, whether they are fond of eating and drinking *to excess* and given to sedentary living or they are fond of exercise and labour'.

A similar sentiment on the relationship of the environment to life was expressed by Guru Nanak (1469-1539), when he said: '*Pawan guru, pani pita, mata dhart muhat, divis raat doi daii daia, khele sagal jagat'*. (Air is like God, water is the father and earth is the mother. It is through the harmonious interaction of all these three vital ingredients that the whole universe is being sustained).

AIR POLLUTION

An adult can survive without food for three weeks, without water for three days but not more than three minutes without air. Such is the importance of fresh air to life.

The last fifty years have seen a rapid growth in industry, an ever-increasing number of transport vehicles and overcrowding of urban populations. The exhaust from chemical factories, thermal power stations, motor vehicles and generator sets have thrown a large number of pollutants into the environment. These have proved harmful to the human population through the polluted food eaten, the polluted air breathed in and contact of the chemicals with the skin and the eyes. The toxins in the polluted air mostly affect the lungs, skin, eyes and kidneys, and are carcinogenic but the cardiovascular system is also affected indirectly or directly by the harmful elements in the polluted air.

Carbon Monoxide (CO) and the Cardiovascular System

The combining power of CO with haemoglobin is 210 times more than oxygen (O). The sources of CO are cigarette smoking, vehicular emissions and passive smoking. When carbon monoxide enters the blood, it immediately displaces the oxygen and mixes with haemoglobin to result in carboxyhaemoglobin which results in damage to all the vital organs. The sufferer turns blue, gets asphyxia and as oxygen does not reach the vital organs like the heart and the brain, these may suffer irreversible damage that proves fatal if the carbon monoxide is not immediately replaced with oxygen. Children and elderly people are more vulnerable to this effect. Smokers carry 10-20 per cent carboxyhaemoglobin, depending upon the number of cigarettes smoked. Symptoms like headache, dizziness, confusion, lassitude and severe breathlessness precede death. Pollution of air due to carbon monoxide also increases the occurrence of congestive heart failure in the elderly. Preventive strategies against morbidity and mortality from carbon monoxide poisoning should be targetted against vehicular exhaust by strict legislation and by introducing anti-smoking measures at large.

Cigarette Smoke

Tobacco contains about 1500 toxins, including nicotine as the major one. Among others are carbon monoxide, hydrogen cyanide, methane, formaldehyde and several hydrocarbons. The general health hazards of cigarette smoking are well known—chronic bronchitis, lung cancer, cancer of the voice-box, stomach, urinary bladder and

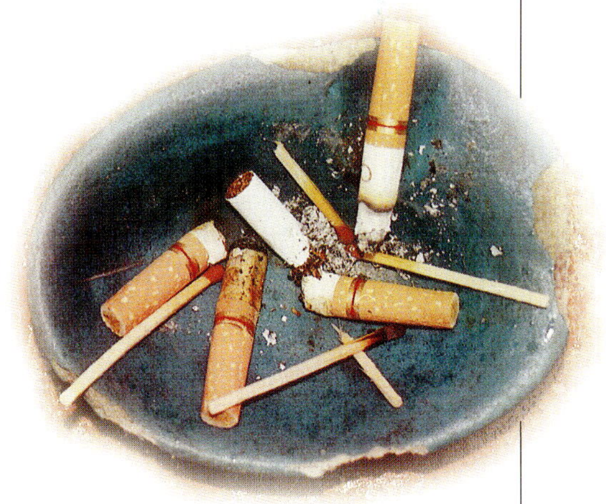

cervix. The cardiovascular harmful effects of smoking include increased pulse rate, spasm of the coronary arteries, angina, myocardial infarction, peripheral arterial disease (Burger's disease is a painful condition of the legs, often ending in gangrene and loss of limbs). Sudden cardiac death is also more common in smokers. Passive smoking through pollution of atmospheric air by side-stream smoke is responsible for 53,000 deaths annually in the USA. Smoking also results in increased blood fibrinogen levels (clotting factor), blood viscosity (thickness) and polycythemia (increased red corpuseles — all these factors aggravate coronary heart disease. In a study conducted at the All India Institute of Medical Sciences (AIIMS), India, smoking was the major risk factor for myocardial infarction in patients below 40 years of age who were proven to have coronary artery disease in coronary angiographies. As cessation of smoking reverses the harmful effect of smoking, including heart disease, anti-smoking campaigns should be put into practice on a war footing.

Other Air Pollutants

Poor air quality due to various pollutants has the potential for serious adverse health effects on various systems, including the cardiovascular system through perturbances of cellular ecology over long periods of exposure. In one study from Michigan, USA, air pollution with suspended particulate matter was associated with high daily admissions for ischaemic heart disease, specially among the elderly above 65 years of age. Ozone (O_3), which comes from vehicle exhaust, is also related to high daily mortality in summer, as during that season the ozone levels in the air are found to be high, as per a study from London. Ozone has toxic effects on the bronchi and myocardium. Nitrogen dioxide (NO_2), another pollutant from vehicular emission, mostly from diesel engines, may result in pulmonary oedema (excessive fluid

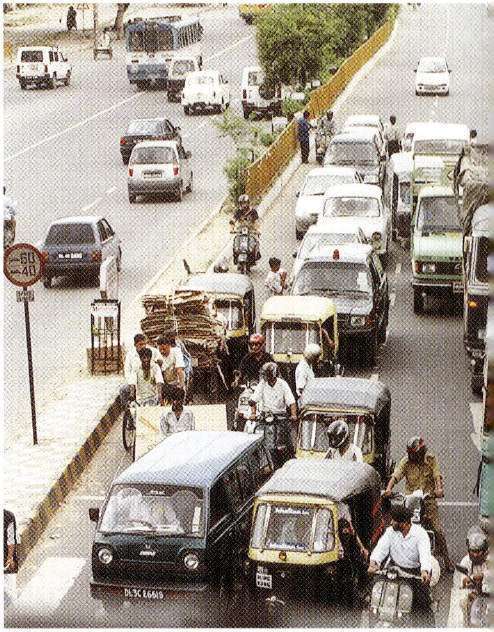

in the lungs) and aggravation of coronary disease. Diesel-driven vehicles are the main source of sulphur dioxide which is responsible for many cardio-pulmonary diseases. Air pollution from sulphur dioxide (SO_2) occurs through coal and wood burnt for fuel, thermal power station exhausts and vehicular emissions, more so diesel

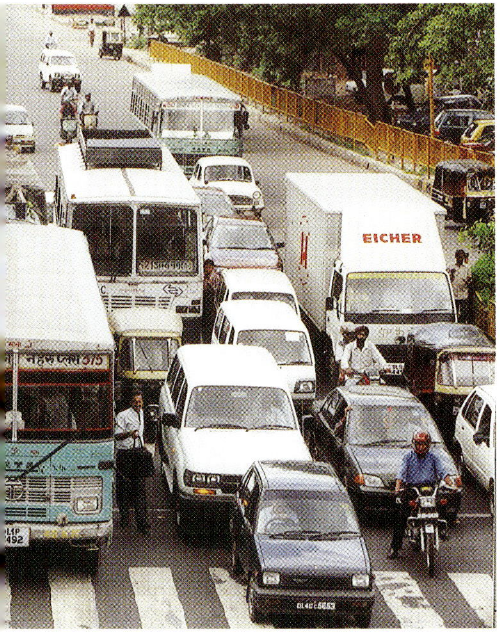

exhaust. Toxic effects of SO_2 include impaired lung function and exercise capacity, higher mortality from neoplasms (abnormal growth of tissue in some part of the body), cardiovascular disease and lung diseases. Air pollution due to lead (Pb) occurs through leaded petrol. Toxic effects of lead pollution include an impaired IQ, development defects in children and, possibly, hypertension. Cadmium has also been reported to be related to the development of hypertension, possibly due to its effect on proximal renal tubules.

Apart from the toxic effects, some air pollutants produce a bad odour and a nauseating feeling, thus indirectly affecting the cardiovascular system through a disturbed heart rate and blood pressure, which, in turn, could aggravate angina, arrhythmias and congestive heart failure or initiate the onset of an acute heart attack.

TEMPERATURE CHANGES

The ideal reading for temperature for a human being is between 20°-25°C / 68°-70°F. Temperature extremes result in high morbidity and mortality from cardiovascular disease due to fluid and electrolyte imbalance at high temperatures, and due to increased peripheral resistance and blood pressure at lower temperatures. In a study from the Netherlands, there was a 57 per cent higher cold-related unexpected mortality at temperatures below 20°C/68°F and an excess of 26 per cent heat-related unexpected mortality at temperatures above 25°C/77°F. This higher mortality with extremes of temperatures was attributed to cardiovascular causes.

NOISE POLLUTION

Chronic exposure of children to the high-level urban traffic noise has been reported to result in higher blood pressures. This effect is reported to be due to the increase in heart rate and peripheral vascular resistance. Environmental noise pollution could thus be a contributing factor to higher prevalence of hypertension amongst city dwellers. Preventive strategies against hypertension must, therefore, make note of this observation and accordingly institute desirable measures, especially during childhood.

Ever-increasing urban migration and rapidly mushrooming industrial units have resulted in grave ecological imbalance due to environmental pollution.

Prevention and Control of Air Pollution

As the sources of air pollution are industrial, vehicular and domestic (indoor), the preventive strategies therefore have to be focussed on at the following levels:

Industrial Air Pollution

This can be controlled by strict legislation recommending the height of chimneys and provision of

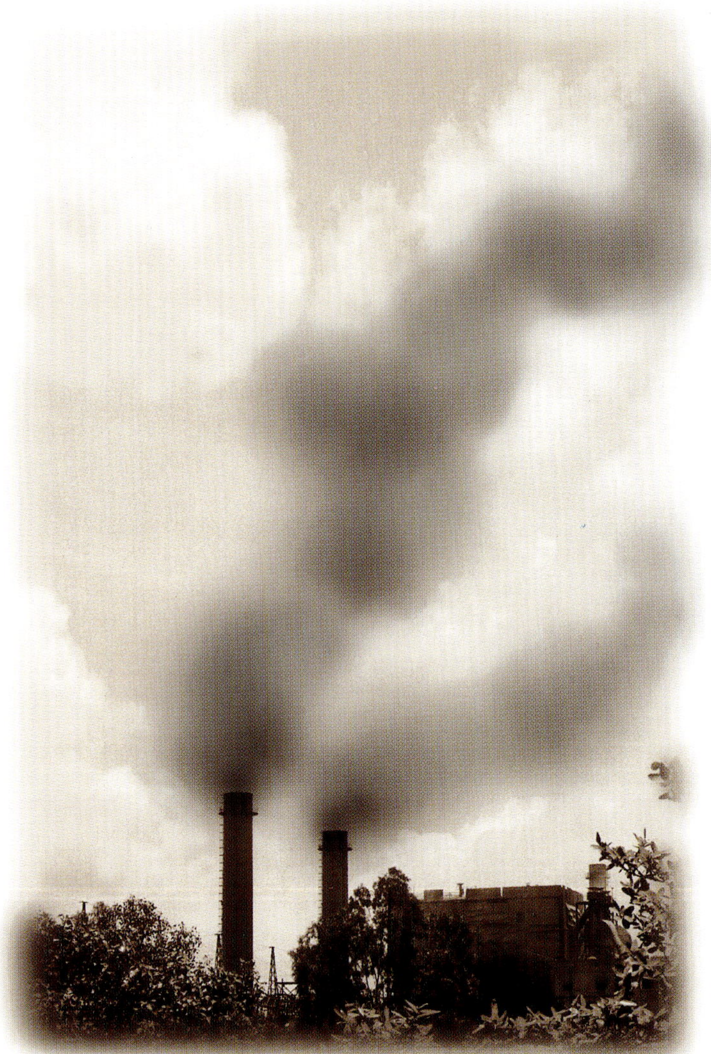

industrial filters for the exhaust that is produced in thermal power stations and other industries using coal, diesel, wood, kerosene or other fuels as energy sources. Industrial units using such fuel should not be allowed to operate in residential areas. Knowledge of protective devices against chemical warfare may be extended in planning of preventive strategies against urban air pollution.

Vehicular Pollution

In some countries, common transport media still comprise cycles, two or three-wheelers and rickshaws. A large number of people walk to their places of work. These city dwellers are prone to the maximum adverse effects of air pollution from vehicular traffic run on diesel and leaded petrol. A periodic check of the vehicles and punishment for the defaulters is the only solution to control vehicular air pollution.

Domestic Pollution

Passive inhalation of smoke from cigarettes and stoves, and the use of generator sets run on kerosene, petrol or diesel are the sources of indoor air pollution. Strongly discouraging cigarette smoking, use of electric inverters in place of generators, keeping generator sets at higher levels and providing adequate air filters are recommended for control of indoor pollution.

Deforestation of the rural areas surrounding large cities to provide houses for the ever-increasing urban migration has disturbed the ecology and health relationship between the fauna and flora and human population. Growing of more trees will restore this healthy relationship, thereby preventing many disorders caused by air pollution.

If adequate preventive measures against air pollution are not thought of and put into practice *now,* then even breathing in certain highly polluted areas may become lethal to health.

> **A** *higher standard of living must be achieved without causing ecological imbalance and despoiling nature of its beauty, freshness and purity essential to our lives.*

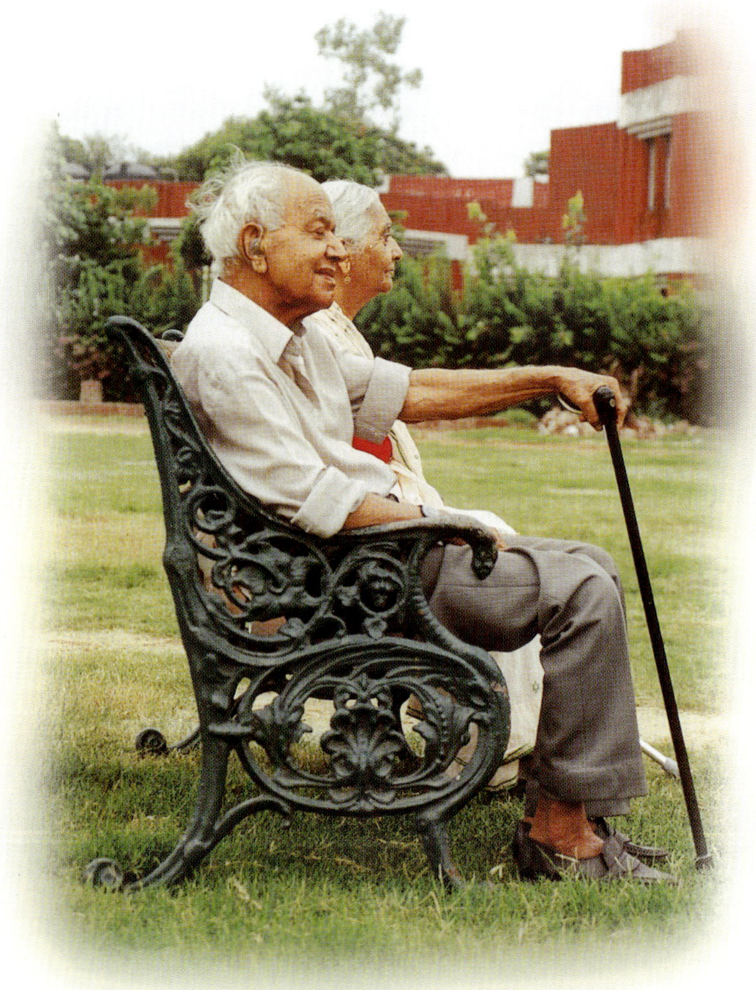

6. Heart Care of the Elderly

Rapid scientific developments in medical science, specially over the last fifty years, have, to a large extent, contributed to improving the quality of life and lengthening the lifespan. This has resulted in more people reaching old age and suffering from heart disease, high blood pressure and cancer. Intervention procedures like balloon angioplasty, laser, stents, coils and pacemakers have given heart patients a new lease of life and enhanced their quality of life. The wonders of heart, lung, kidney, liver and other organ transplants have enabled many people to live productive lives for a longer time than was ever thought possible in the past.

Age has more to do with our attitudes and thoughts than biological aging. As G. Edward put it: *'It is not by the grey of the hair that one knows the age of the heart.'* The setting sun of retirement brings with it several psycho-social, personal and health-related problems. Most countries of the world are being governed by a head of state beyond 60 years of age. Depending upon the average life expectancy, the retirement age is variable between 55 years and 75 years in various countries; it is also job related, being the lowest in the military services and highest in the judiciary.

The fact of an individual reaching the age of retirement is obviously due to reasonably good health. Having survived beyond the fifth or sixth decade of life, the diseases that one is likely to encounter are those of the cardiovascular system and cancer. Heart diseases and strokes are the commonest killers as well as responsible for disability in the aged.

'We are as old as our arteries', is an old saying. Heart attacks and brain attacks (strokes) being responsible for maximum deaths and disability in the elderly, the modern version of the above quotation could perhaps be rephrased to read: *'We are as old as our coronary and cerebral arteries'*.

The grey zone of 60-65 years may be considered the zone of post-retirement beyond which people are placed in the category of senior citizens. According to WHO calculations, by the year 2000, there

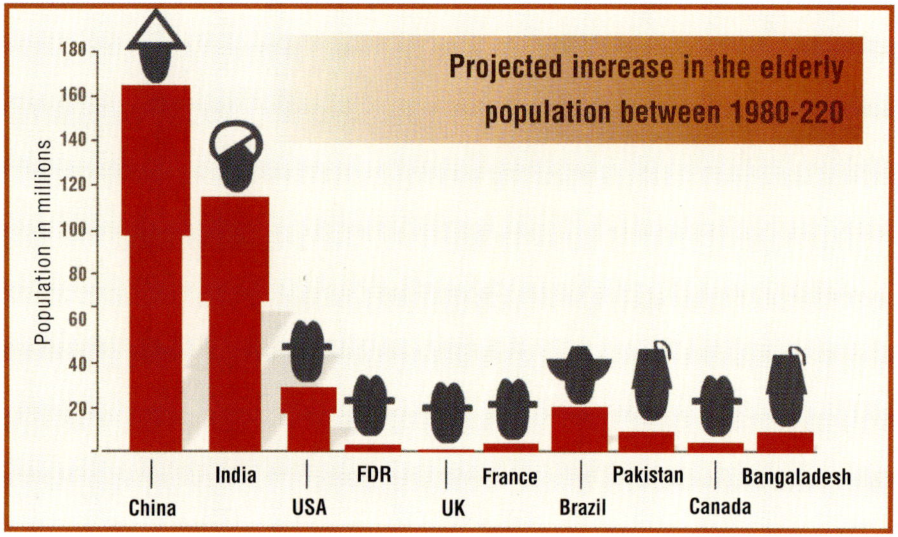

were likely to be 100 million people over the age of 65 in developing countries. These senior citizens would have obviously withstood successfully the tests of infections, to then enter the arena where they would face degenerative disorders. Although old age does not provide immunity from infectious diseases, yet the major cause of mortality and morbidity in the elderly are cancer and cardiovascular diseases.

Cardiovascular Diseases in the Elderly

The main cause of death accounting for geriatric mortality is cardiovascular disease. It accounts for nearly one-third of deaths in the elderly, mainly from coronary disease, stroke and congestive heart failure, the basic process being that of atherosclerosis or narrowing of the arteries that supply pure oxygenated blood to the heart, brain, kidneys, the viscera and the limbs.

Although there are some patients with congenital heart diseases such as aortic stenosis (narrowing) and atrial septal defect (division in the upper two heart cavities), and occasional cases of rheumatic valvular lesions in those aged above 60, yet the commonest cardiovascular problems seen in the elderly are coronary heart disease (heart attacks and angina); hypertension; stroke; arrhythmias requiring pacemakers or drug treatment; congestive heart failure; varicose veins; painful claudication of legs due to atheroscelоritic narrowing of arteries, thereby hampering blood supply specially when more blood is required, such as during walking. Weakening of the walls of large arteries and the aorta also results in sac-like widening of these blood vessels — a disorder called aneurysm. A rupture of one of these dilated blood vessels may result in loss of consciousness, paralytic stroke and even sudden death. Another type of heart disease seen in association with chronic lung disease in the elderly is the condition of chronic corpulmonale — a condition of right heart failure (leg oedema, liver congestion, cyanosis and congested prominent neck veins), which is a result of chronic bronchitis, smoking or prolonged exposure to domestic or industrial smoke and fumes.

Cardiac Care in the Elderly

The elderly should be given a very patient hearing. Minor complaints like, 'not feeling too bright today', and 'profuse undue sweating' could be a manifestation of silent heart attack specially among elderly diabetics, and should not be ignored.

Environmental factors such as sudden changes in temperature, extreme cold or heat have a strong deleterious effect on the cardiovascular function in the elderly; senior citizens have to be protected against such exposures in order to prevent frequent occurrence of aggravation of angina, heart attack, tachyarrhythmias (rapid and at times irregular beating of the heart) and congestive heart failure.

Disease, disability or death of a spouse or a close friend often result in serious disturbances and imbalance in the psychological behaviour of the elderly and this, in turn, aggravates or initiates serious cardiac malfunction. Death within a few months of the demise of the spouse is not uncommon among senior citizens.

Special Treatment Considerations for the Elderly

While most drugs, devices and surgical procedures used for cardiac patients in general can also be used and are being used successfully in the elderly too, certain therapeutic precautions are worth considering:

- Drug clearance is delayed by the kidney and liver in the elderly, so dosages of various drugs should be modified accordingly in amount and frequency of administration.

- The elderly as such are hypo-kinetic (slow in their movements, in their responses and reactions), so sedatives and tranquillisers should be given in a smaller dosage and under careful monitoring.

- It is preferable to give the least number of drugs with a smaller dosage for short periods.

■ Except in emergency situations like myocardial infarction complicated with shock or serious arrhythmias where ICCU (Intensive Cardiac Care Unit) treatment and monitoring may be mandatory, the elderly should preferably be treated at home. If hospitalisation is necessary, a close relative should be permitted to stay with the aged patient.

■ While the elderly are not denied any cardiac operation, their other systems like lung function, kidney status, cerebrovascular status and condition of their prostate should be carefully examined. A satisfactory functioning of all these systems is necessary for a successful outcome of any heart operation.

■ Non-cardiac surgery is often needed: surgery of the prostate, cataract, gall bladder, uterus, joint replacements and dental extractions. It is important to ascertain that the patient's blood pressure is within the normal range; any arrhythmia should be treated adequately, and unless it is a dire emergency, routine operations should be postponed until three months after a heart attack. For a patient with an advanced degree of heart block, a temporary pacemaker may be necessary before the patient goes for a major surgery under general anaesthesia. In rare cases if a patient has severe angina and a coronary angiography shows one or more coronary arteries to be significantly diseased, this patient should be first subjected to myocardial revascularisation by either ballooning angioplasty or bypass surgery before any major non-cardiac surgery is undertaken.

■ When using drugs in the elderly for the treatment of hypertension, heart failure or arrhythmias, close monitoring is needed to watch out for side-effects which may impair their quality of life like constipation, postural giddiness (due to postural hypotension—low blood pressure), muscle weakness (hyponatremia and hypokalemia), depression (sedatives) and increased frequency of urination (diuretics), which disturbs their sleep. Drugs should be reduced at the earliest possible and stopped if the clinical situation safely permits.

■ Non-surgical intervention like ballooning angioplasty of the coronary and peripheral arteries and stent implantation may be done in the elderly as successfully as in other patients.

■ A large number of the elderly have extended their lifespan by years with the help of a pacemaker. This can be given at any age after ensuring that the renal and cerebral status of the patient is satisfactory and there is no evidence of malignancy. Implantable Cardioverter Defibrillators (ICD) are now available, which automatically detect both fast and slow arrhythmias, and are accordingly chosen to either give an electric shock to terminate the otherwise fatal arrhythmia (ventricular fibrillation) or work as a pacemaker to restart the normal heart rhythm in cases of complete heart blocks. These devices have proved very useful in survivors of sudden cardiac death victims — that is those who have been resuscitated successfully after a cardiac arrest.

■ Cure from cardiac disease may not be possible in all elderly cardiac patients, so the aim should be to make the best use of their limited cardiac capacity to enable them to

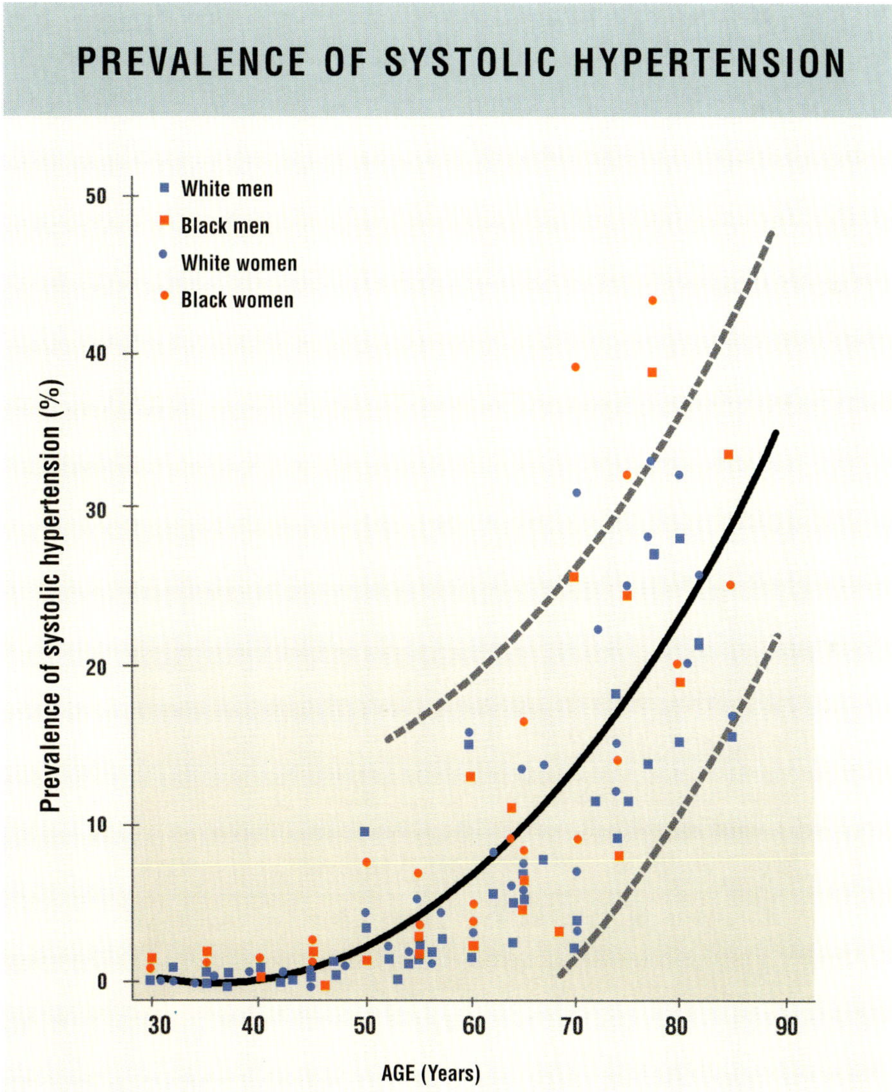

enjoy the optimum quality of life in their remaining years. Interventions and modifications in dietary and living habits may be suggested with due care. Mild to moderately regulated physical exercises should be encouraged but strenuous exercises should be avoided.

Sex in Elderly Heart Patients

It is said: *'Man is as old as he feels and woman as old as she looks.'* A perfect mutual interspouse understanding goes a long way to accomplish the desired sexual needs. However the elderly afflicted with heart disease have to observe certain precautions:

- After a heart attack, a patient can resume sex only when there is no anginal pain or breathlessness during daily routine activities.

- Those with chronic angina should take a nitrate tablet sublingually (under the tongue) before the act.

- Sex should be avoided for about an hour after a meal.

- After a bypass surgery, sex may be resumed as soon as the surgical aches and pains are over and there is no angina on usual exertion.

- The sex potency medicine Viagra should not be taken by those heart patients who are using nitrates in any form.

Prevention of Cardiovascular Disease in the Elderly

General preventive measures such as regular physical exercise, control of hypertension by non-drug means and use of drugs, avoidance of smoking, control of blood lipids by drugs and dietary measures, and mental relaxation with meditation, yoga and music are applicable to the elderly as well. Even when started in later years, these measures have been shown to regress atherosclerosis and prevent or postpone any occurrence of cardiac events.

In an attempt to cure hypertension or heart disease in the elderly, the physician should not injudiciously use various drugs and devices without looking into the overall outcome of these methods of treatment. Any therapeutic measure used in the elderly must not result in deterioration in his/her quality of life at the cost of a few added years. While *cure* from heart disease in the elderly may not be possible for all, *care* of the elderly with a heart disease is certainly possible.

Old age is not the end of the drama of life but only another episode with a new set-up and some changes in the orchestra and the stage. Several historic contributions in the field of arts, education and culture have come from people well into their 'twilight' years. So a disciplined and well-adhered-to routine can prove these lines to be true: '*To be seventy years young is far more cheerful and hopeful than to be forty years old.*'

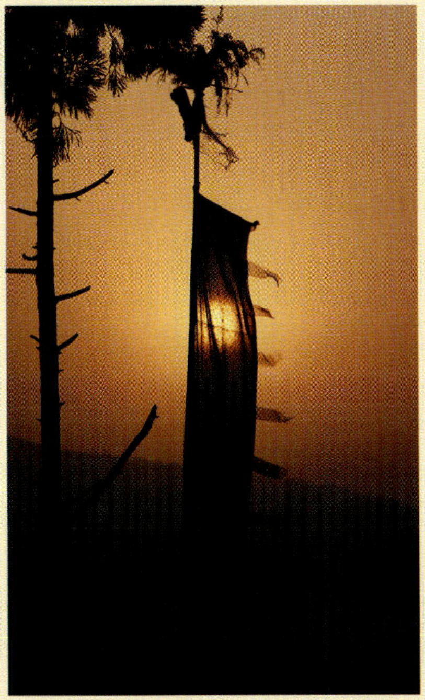

It is too late! Ah nothing is too late,
till the tired heart shall cease to palpitate.
Cato learned Greek at eighty; Sophocles,
wrote his grand Oedipus, and Simondes
bore off the prize of verse from his compeers
when each had numbered more than four score years.
Chaucer at Woodstock with the nightingales,
at sixty wrote the Canterbury Tales;
Goethe at Weimar, toiling to the last,
completed Faust when eighty years were past.
These are indeed exceptions; but they show
how far the gulf-stream of our youth may flow
into the Arctic regions of our lives . . .
for age is opportunity no less
than youth itself, though in another dress,
and as the evening twilight fades away
the sky is filled with stars, invisible by day.

—Longfellow, Morituri Salutamus 1.238

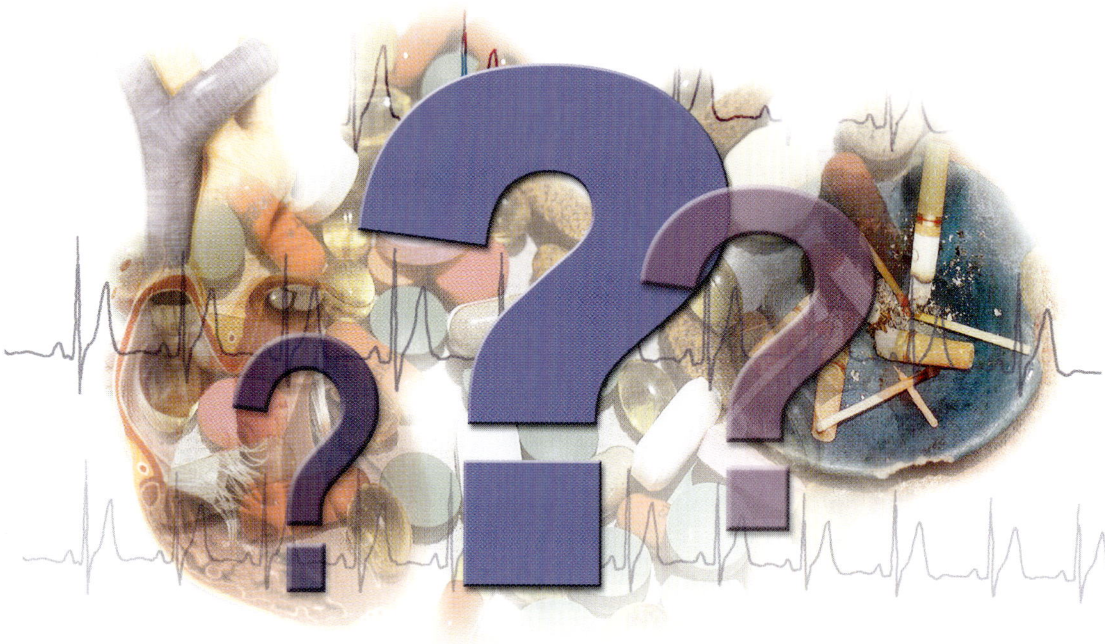

7. Commonly Asked Questions and Answers

In my practice of cardiology over the last 30 years, I have been asked all manner of questions on dangers to the heart, the kind of lifestyle to follow, diagnosis methods, types of treatments, effects of those treatments and reassurances about recurrence of problems. When a patient goes to a cardiologist, he is thoroughly examined through a series of detailed questions. A patient's attendant has his own queries and anxieties.

- Why a TMT and not angiography for precise diagnosis?
- Why not an MRI instead of CT Scan or Thallium test?
- Will there be non-drug treatment or treatment with drugs? Or devices or surgery?

If drugs, then what drugs, as unlike the good old days when there was only one quinine for malaria and chloromycetin for typhoid, these days several drug alternatives are available for one disease, and specially for those where the exact cause of the disease is not known, like heart attacks and high blood pressure. With the strong effect of the media, both print and electronic, and the drug pamphlets available with each drug, there are more questions about the dosages and side-effects of various drugs for which the physician has to remain ever updated. When any devices such as ballooning and stents are used, again there are questions regarding their efficacy, longevity, chances of recurrence of disease in spite of devices and the cost of treatment. The same holds true for various surgical procedures advised for heart disease. Questions on diet,

Q. What actually happens during a heart attack?

A. The heart is the vital organ which supplies oxygen and nutrition to the entire body to sustain life. To work efficiently and non stop, the heart gets its food and fuel through oxygenated blood via three main coronary arteries which sit like a crown (*corona* in Greek means crown) at the top of the heart. If any interruption occurs in this blood supply either due to a blocked artery or temporary narrowing due to a spasm, the heart suffers an 'attack'. The patient complains of severe chest discomfort, chest pain or a heavy pressure in the chest with profuse sweating, nausea and at times, vomiting. The chest discomfort usually lasts for more than 30 minutes.

Q. What are the other reasons for chest pain?

A. Gall bladder stones or gall bladder infection (cholecystitis), spasm or infection of the foodpipe, a stomach ulcer, herpes of the chest wall, pleurisy, cervical spondylosis, inflammation of the heart covering (pericarditis) and a tear (dissection) in the aorta (the major outlet of the heart) are some of the conditions that result in chest pain akin to a heart attack.

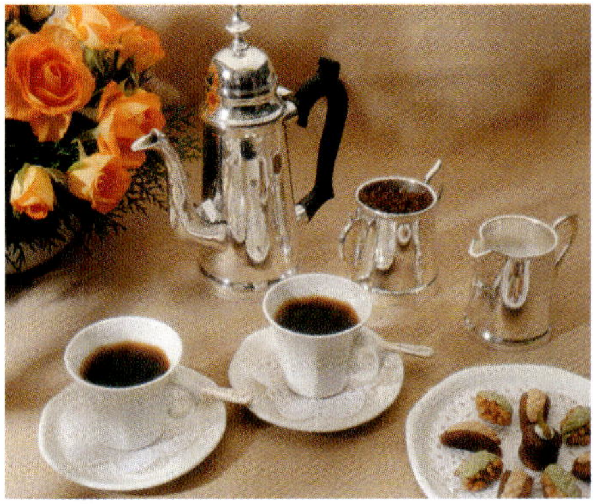

physical exercise and role of the mind and yoga in heart care are often-asked other questions which cannot be simply brushed aside and have to be answered by the doctors as part of holistic heart care and total well-being of their patients.

It is with this background that I felt that some of the commonly asked questions should be addressed directly.

Q. Does chest pain always mean a heart attack?

A. Although heart attack, often synonymous with angina and myocardial infarction (due to coronary artery disease), is an important and serious cause of chest pain, other heart defects such as defects in the heart valves and even high blood pressure can give rise to chest pain.

Q. What is normal blood pressure?

A. As we grow from birth to adulthood, the blood pressure also increases as per the body requirements to maintain adequate circulation for the body mass. From about 60/40 mm Hg at birth, it rises to the average figure of 120/80 mm Hg in the adult. Except in some isolated tribal populations in the world where blood pressure does not rise further after the adulthood pressure has been reached, in most other populations, blood pressure rises with age. It is now universally agreed that readings less than 140/90 mm Hg may be considered as normal and those beyond this are labelled as high blood pressure or hypertension.

Q. Does one reading of 140/90 mm Hg or above mean that a person is suffering from high blood pressure?

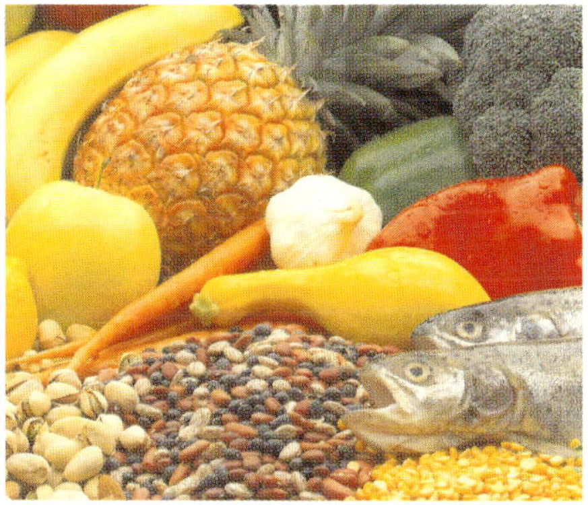

A. No. There is a marked variability in blood pressure depending upon the person's mental state, physical activity and the type of food taken (excess coffee, tea and alcohol tend to increase pressure). At least three blood pressure readings should be taken on different days to ascertain the reading of 140/90 mm Hg or above before starting the treatment, except when the first reading itself is very high, such as beyond 180/100.

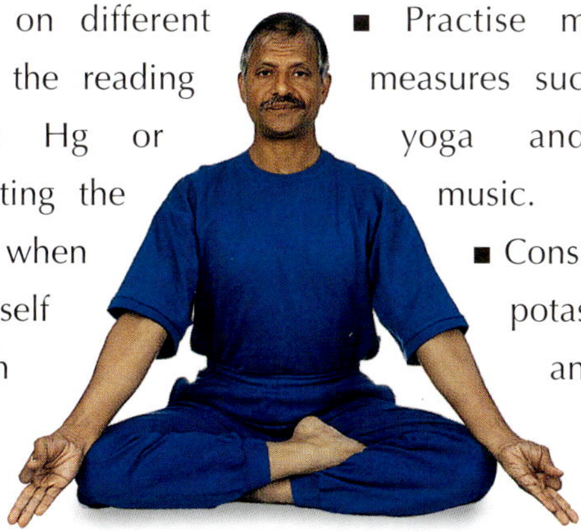

Then immediate treatment is given and further investigations are carried out to find the cause and severity of the disease.

Q. Are there any preventive measures against high blood pressure?

A. Many studies and the World Health Organisation (WHO) have recommended the following measures for prevention of primary hypertension:

- Avoid being overweight and reduce weight if obese.
- Practise mental relaxation measures such as meditation, yoga and listening to music.
- Consume a diet rich in potassium (vegetables and fruits).
- Minimise salt (sodium) intake.

Q. How does one make sure that the chest pain in a particular case is due to heart attack?

A. Severe chest discomfort and pain, mostly in the mid-chest or the left side, radiating to the jaws, back or arms — on the left side more than the right — pain which increases on exertion and is relieved at rest, are all symptoms highly suggestive of *effort angina*. If this condition occurs at rest but is short-lasting, it is called *angina at rest* or *unstable angina*; if this occurs at rest and lasts for more than 30 minutes, and is accompanied by profuse sweating, nausea and, at times, vomiting, it points to a diagnosis of heart attack (myocardial infarction). An ECG, blood enzyme tests, Echo and coronary angiography tests can confirm the diagnosis.

- Reduce alcohol consumption to less than 60 ml of whisky daily or its equivalent of two glasses of beer or wine.
- Do regular physical exercise.

Q. What do the words 'heart attack' mean?

A. A sudden occurrence of an event which has an adverse effect on the normal functioning of the heart is called a heart attack. It is generally the result of a blocked coronary artery.

Q. What is the basic cause for a heart attack?

A. The basic process that results in narrowing and clogging of coronary arteries is called *atherosclerosis.* Although the root cause of this process is unknown the **(i)** presence of high blood levels of cholesterol, **(ii)** high blood pressure, **(iii)** cigarette smoking, **(iv)** lack of physical exercise and **(v)** facing repetitive emotional stresses and strains in a hostile environment are some of the known risk factors that initiate and aggravate atherosclerosis which ultimately results in a heart attack.

There is some research evidence emerging that inflammation of the arterial intima, specially the endothelial layer, due to some chemical (oxydized LDL) or infective agent (chlamydia pneumonae) could also be contributing in the genesis, progression or sudden ulceration of the atheroscleratic plaque, thus causing an acute coronary event (heart attack).

Q. What is low blood pressure?

A. Low blood pressure is not a disease and when an exceptionally low reading is found in a person, one should look for the underlying cause such as severe dehydration, reaction to a drug or a silent heart attack which is common among diabetics.

Q. Can atherosclerosis be prevented or made to regress if already formed?

A. There is experimental, clinical and angiographic evidence to support the view that atherosclerosis may be regressed or postponed by:

- Lowering blood lipids such as cholesterol, LDL (Low Density Liproprotein) and triglycerides.
- Avoiding cigarette smoking.
- Keeping the blood pressure reading below 140/90 mm Hg.
- Avoiding sedentary living habits.
- Doing regular physical exercise. Physical exercise increases blood

levels of nitric oxide, a substance found to be anti-atherosclerotic and cardio-protective.

- Consuming a diet rich in vegetables, nuts, fruits and coarse grains. Processed foods, milk and dairy products and red meat which are rich sources of harmful saturated fats like cholesterol, LDL and sodium salts, and poor in potassium and fibre should be avoided.

Q. Does overweight or obesity play any role in heart attack?

A. It has been observed that people who are overweight, that is, those with BMI (Body Mass Index = Weight in Kgs divided by height in meters^2) above 27, have high levels of blood cholesterol and triglycerides, low HDL (High Density Lipoprotein) which is the good, heart-friendly cholesterol and higher blood pressures—all these being the risk factors for heart attacks.

Q. Do most patients of high blood pressure (primary hypertension) need lifelong therapy?

A. In patients with mild hypertension (blood pressure of 140-159/ 80-90 mm Hg, lifestyle modifications such as **(i)** reduction in body weight if overweight, **(ii)** doing regular physical exercise, **(iii)** reducing salt and alcohol consumption, **(iv)** inculcating the habit of mental relaxation through meditation, music and yoga help in normalising blood pressure. Even in those with high blood pressures beyond 160/100 mm Hg, these measures help in reducing drug requirements. Lifelong drug therapy may not be necessary. If the treatment is started early and lifestyle measures are strictly adhered to, many patients may not need any medicine.

Interestingly weight reduction by dietary control and regular exercise normalises these abnormalities.

Q. What should one do in the event of a heart attack?

A. Avoid creating panic. Call for medical help and take the patient to a nearby centre which has facilities to treat patients with acute heart attack.

While waiting for medical help, give the patient a tablet of aspirin to chew (avoid in a case of stomach ulcer or other bleeding disorder), a tranquilliser or a sedative. Avoid overcrowding around the patient. Administering a nitrate tablet, unlike in patients of chronic angina, usually *does not* help in a patient with acute heart attack and should *not* be repeated if there is no relief with the already-given one tablet, as this may result in a serious fall in blood pressure.

Once in the hospital, the doctor will discuss the mode of treatment and its various medical and financial implications. The attendant should carefully understand and discuss all these points instead of merely saying, 'Doctor, you are the best judge; do whatever you think best for the patient'. The doctor, of course, is the judge. But due to the serious nature of the disease or the interventions done to treat the disease, if some untoward complication occurs, the doctor should not be unnecessarily held resonsible due to an initial lack of proper communication between the doctor and the patient and his attendants.

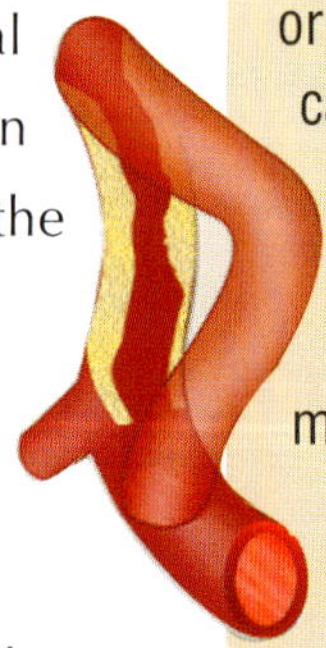

Q. Are bypass and ballooning permanent cures?

A. Neither ballooning nor bypass surgery is really a permanent cure. One should take adequate steps to avoid recurrence of a heart attack even after these procedures have been done. These measures include:

- Control blood pressure and blood lipids through dietary measures or drugs.
- Avoid cigarette smoking.
- Do regular physical exercise.
- Control body weight.

Q. Can bypass surgery be done on a beating heart?

A. Normally the heart is put out of circulation and its beating stopped for a little while to help the surgeon to do the 'plumbing' to clear the blocks and place the bypass grafts on a quiet non-beating heart. During this time the blood circulation for the entire body is taken over by the heart lung machine (cardio-pulmonary bypass). These days, however, in certain cases with a minimal number of blocks in one or two arteries, bypass surgery can be done without using the heart-lung machine through smaller cuts in the chest on a beating heart through minimally invasive surgery called MID CAB surgery or 'Off Pump' surgery.

Q. What are the ballooning procedures and how do these help a heart patient?

A. Ballooning or angioplasty as it is called in interventional cardiology is the procedure whereby a blocked blood vessel is opened with the help of an expandable balloon made of a special material to withstand inflation pressures of upto 10-15 atmospheres. Depending upon the organ or system of which the blood

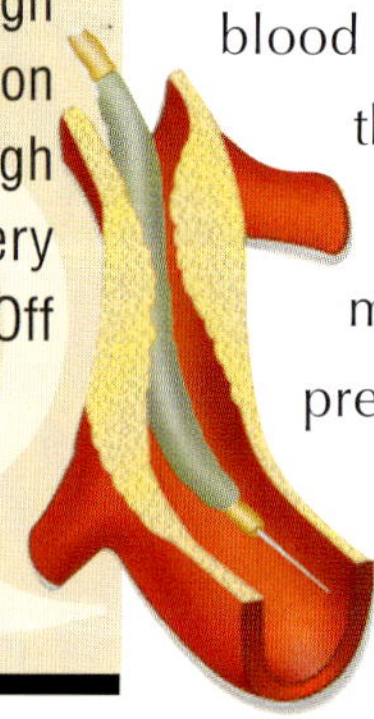

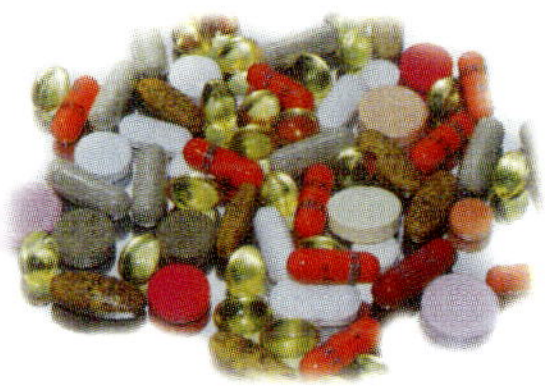

vessels are being opened, the procedure goes by that name such as coronary angioplasty (angina and heart attacks), renal angioplasty (kidney), aorta, carotid (for strokes) and peripheral angioplasty (for limbs), to name a few. In patients who have had a bypass surgery and whose veins get blocked after five to ten years of the bypass, ballooning can be done in the blocked veins too.

Q. Why is alcohol harmful?

A. While small amounts of alcohol do not harm and may even be beneficial both for cordial social interaction and relaxation, heavy alcohol consumption of more than two ounces of whisky in a day or its equivalent of two glasses of beer or two glasses of wine is harmful not only for the liver and stomach but also for the heart as it results in higher blood pressure and harmful blood fats which are the risk factors for heart attacks. Heavy drinking is also responsible for social problems such as traffic accidents, deaths, divorces, absence from work, homicides . . .

Q. What are *stents* and which patients need them?

A. After opening the blocked vessels with the help of ballooning, in about 30% patients, the block occurs again (restenosis) within a few months, sometimes even within weeks, thus requiring another ballooning procedure. In order to avoid this from happening, fine coils made of special material are inserted at the site of the obstructions after opening them with balloons. These tiny coils measuring from a few millimetres to a few centimetres in size, depending upon the size of the blocks, are called *stents*. Use of stents has not totally eliminated the process of restenosis but significantly reduced it to below 10%.

Q. Is ballooning useful for other heart patients apart from those with angina and heart attacks?

A. Ballooning is used for children who are born with structural defects in their heart (congenital heart disease). These defects are mainly of three types:

1. Where pure (oxygenated) blood mixes with the impure blood due to holes or defects in the heart chambers

2. Narrow heart valves or vessels

3. Mixed variety with both holes and obstructions

Ballooning is helpful in patients with narrow valves (aortic and pulmonary stenosis) or vessels — (like the congenital narrowing of the aorta). Similarly ballooning is now the preferred treatment for mitral stenosis (narrowing of the valve between the left atrium and the left ventricle), the commonest heart valve disease in our country due to rheumatic fever (mitral balloon valvotomy). Ballooning has thus replaced heart surgery, including open heart surgery, in most such situations.

Q. What role do our lifestyles play in our well-being in general and heart care in particular?

A. Lifestyles means the system and styles we follow in our day-to-day living, such as the surroundings or the environment we live in, the air we breathe, the food we eat and the fluids we drink. Environmental pollution with exhausts from industrial chimneys and road transport adversely affects our eyes, skin, lungs, brain and heart. Noise also affects our hearing, mental functions and blood pressure. While overweight, diabetes, high blood cholesterol, heart attacks and high blood pressure are due to faulty eating and drinking habits, smoking causes cancer of the lungs and voice box, bronchitis and blood vessel diseases. The dioxides of sulphur and nitrogen, carbon monoxide and the particulate matter in vehicular exhaust are injurious to the heart and circulatory system.

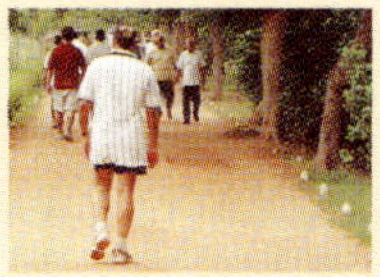
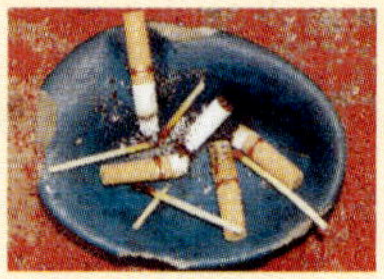
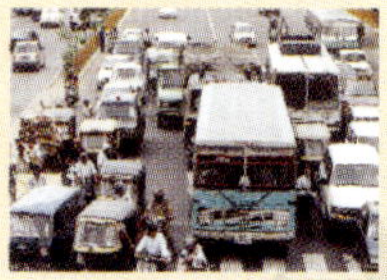
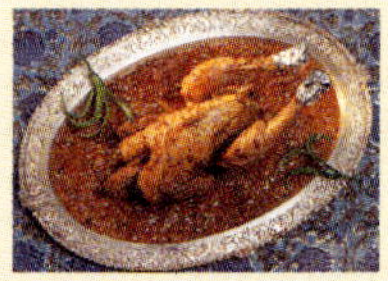

Q. What is the role of bypass surgery at present in the treatment of heart disease?

A. In a bypass operation, a blocked coronary artery is bypassed by using, most often, one of the leg veins (sephenous vein) or an artery from the chest wall (internal mammary artery), although some other arteries like the radial from the hand or some other from the abdomen may also be used. This procedure restores the blood supply to the heart muscle by bypassing the blocked native coronary arteries. The arterial conduits are longer lasting than veins which tend to get narrow after five to ten years, thus needing another bypass or ballooning procedure. Most cases which in

Q. Does the mind play a role in heart care?

A. It is a common observation based on experimental, clinical and population studies that animals kept under a stressful state in a hostile environment tend to have higher blood pressure, and persons working in challenging, tense and stressful situations have higher incidence of high blood pressure, irregular heart rhythms and other related cardiovascular ailments. Stress plays a major role on the working of all the body organs, including the brain, stomach, intestines and heart. Mental relaxation through practice of yoga, meditation, music, relaxing indoor games and physical exercise helps in preserving and promoting the well-being of the heart by keeping the heart rate, rhythm and blood pressure under control, and thereby preventing heart attacks.

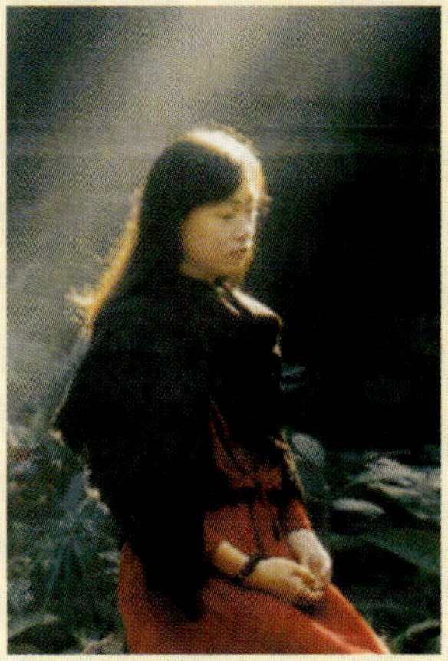

earlier times used to be subjected to open heart bypass surgery, can these days be helped by the non-surgical procedure of ballooning with or without stenting.

Bypass surgery, however, continues to be the choice treatment in diabetics and patients who have multiple blocks at more than three or four sites. Multiple ballooning with stenting can be done but it increases the cost which often works out higher than that for bypass surgery.

Q. Is there anything else apart from balloons and bypass to help victims of heart attack?

A. In some patients where the arteries are very small, the disease is widespread and blocks are present in more peripheral segments of the arteries, neither ballooning nor bypass surgery is of much help. The only way in which blood circulation may be improved to the heart in such patients is to make several small channels in the heart muscle of the left ventricle so that the oxygenated blood seeps directly into the muscle (popularly called 'snake heart' operation as this is the pattern in snakes). In days gone by, these channels were made by open heart surgery either mechanically or through lasers but now the procedure can be done without surgery by inserting a special catheter device through the groin artery. This is called Percutaneous

Trans-Myocardial Revascularisation (PTMR).

Q. When are the pacemakers and defibrillators used in the treatment of heart disease?

A. A pacemaker is a small device used to maintain adequate heart rate in patients with very slow rates — usually less than 40 per minute — and having transient attacks of unconsciousness (synocopal attacks). These are battery-run devices generally placed in the chest wall; the batteries last for more than 10 years and sometimes even for a lifetime. Pacemakers have saved many lives and improved the quality of living in many others.

A defibrillator is a device used to treat patients with fast and often irregular heart rhythms with electrical means (cardioversion). It is a life-saving device for heart patients. Automatic Implantable Cardiovertor Defibrillators (ICDs) implanted in high risk patients of serious arrhythmias have saved many heart patients from sudden cardiac death. Survivors of sudden cardiac death by Cardiopulmonary Resuscitation (CPR) are candidates for implanting such defibrillator-pacemaker devices.

Q. Is there anything else beyond ballooning, bypass and Percutaneous Trans-Myocardial Revascularisation (PTMR) for patients with heart disease?

A. Patients with an end-stage heart disease are not responsive to surgical or interventional techniques. However, with the well-preserved functioning of other organs, they can undergo heart replacement by miniatured artificial (mechanical) hearts, as conventional heart transplant surgery is not the answer due to several reasons

Q. How does food affect the heart?

A. It is not only the quantity and the quality of food we eat but also the environment in which we eat, which has a significant impact on the heart. Eating delicious food in a hostile environment may not give as much satisfaction as eating simple food amidst jovial company, even in simple surroundings.

This observation is based on scientific studies done on the gastric

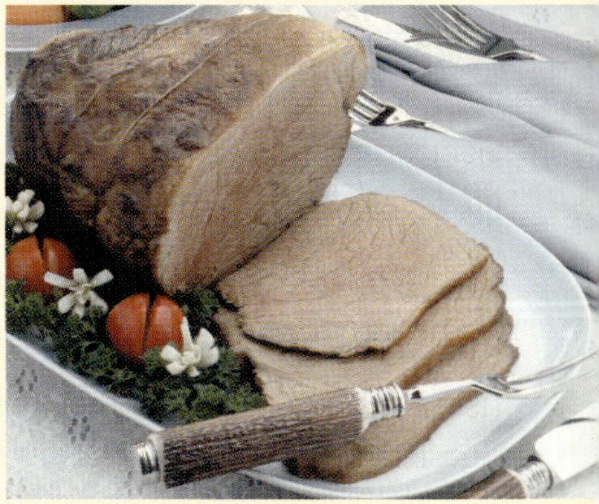

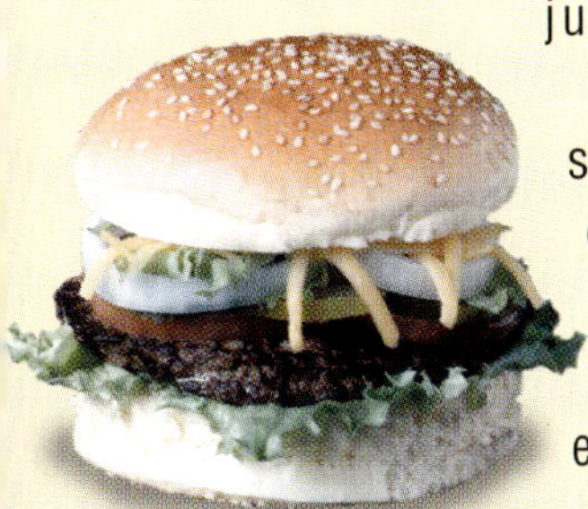

juices and hormones secreted in our body in response to the environmental factors prevalent at the time of eating. What affects the heart adversely is the habit of (i) overeating, (ii) consuming too much saturated fat of animal origin (meat, milk and dairy products), (iii) excessive alcohol consumption and (iv) less intake of vegetables, fresh fruits, and nuts as these are the rich sources of antioxidants, fibre and certain elements of vitamins of the B group which are cardio-protective. Overeating leads to overweight and increases blood cholesterol and blood pressure which are the risk factors for heart attacks. Gooseberries *(amlas)*, onions, garlic

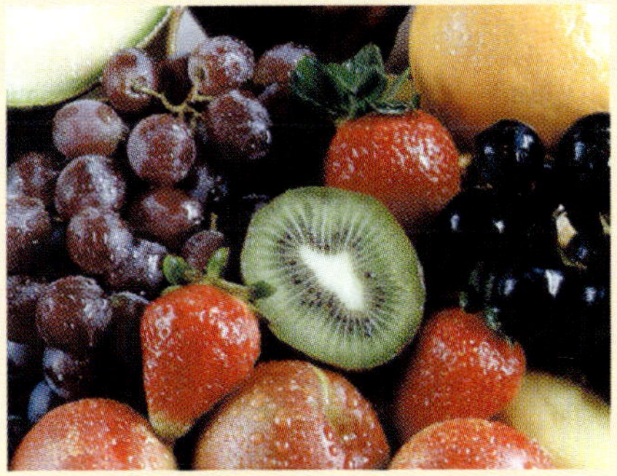

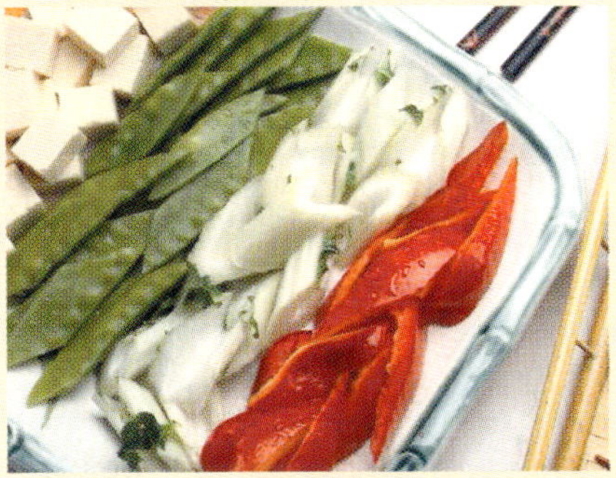

and grapes are heart-friendly dietary items by virtue of their being rich sources of cardio-protective agents such as flavenoids and antioxidants which help in counteracting the harmful effects of free radicals.

including the uncertainty of donors, implications of rejections and lifelong anti-rejection drug therapy. The 21st century is going to witness a lot of exciting research in the field of gene therapy for new blood vessel formation and use of mechanical hearts.

Q. How does smoking affect the heart?

A. Cigarette smoking and tobacco use in other forms are not only injurious to health in general, but may be lethal for the heart too. While tobacco chewing results in ulcers and cancer of the mouth, lips and the inner parts of the cheeks, cigarette smoking enhances the narrowing of arteries by atherosclerosis and spasm, resulting in angina and heart attacks. The other bad effects of smoking are bronchitis and cancer of the voice box, lungs, urinary bladder and cervix. The

Q. What is rheumatic fever and how does it affect the heart?

A. Rheumatic fever generally occurs in childhood during school-going age as a consequence of bacterial (streptococcal) sore throat. It manifests as joint pains (arthralgia) or painful swelling (arthritis) of major joints like elbows, wrists, knees and ankles; fever and malaise, preceded by a sore throat. In many cases it affects the heart, resulting in leaky valves and heart failure. If not treated in the initial stages with antibiotics, aspirin or cortisone (steroids), it may result in permanent damage to the heart valves, requiring ballooning or valve replacement or repair of the damaged valves. Rheumatic fever thus 'licks' the joints but 'bites' the heart.

person sitting around the active smoker also get adversely affected by the exhaled smoke—this goes by the name of *passive smoking.*

Q. How does physical exerise help to keep the heart in good shape?

A. Sedentary living habits make you put on weight and make you less efficient in daily working as your system stays out of tune and muscles, out of practice. Physical exercise, on the other hand, trains the body muscles to perform more efficiently even with less oxygen supply, keeps body weight under control, burns out excess food consumed, corrects elevated blood sugar, blood lipids and blood pressure and is the best means to achieve physical and mental relaxation. This happens through the effect of agents called endorphins which are liberated into the blood stream during physical exercise. In

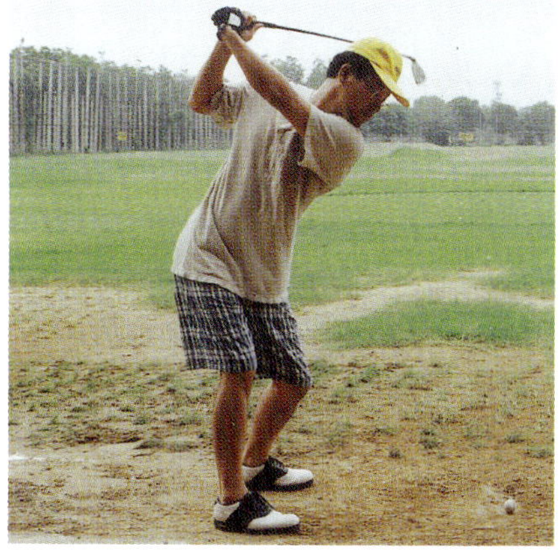

fact regular moderate physical exercise not only helps in prevention of high blood pressure and diabetes but is also the non-drug treatment for these diseases. Recent reseach has demonstrated that several beneficial effects of physical exercise occur through its virtue of increasing the nitric oxide in blood circulation, an agent which is useful

Q. What are the common symptoms that make one suspect that he/she may be suffering from heart disease?

A. The cardinal features that make one suspicious of having heart disease are: chest pain, shortness of breath on exertion or at rest, palpitation, quick fatigue, blackouts or transient attacks of unconsciousness.

At the on set of any one of these symptoms, one should consult the physician who, after an initial assessment, may like to consult a cardiologist. It is important to remember that being overweight, anaemic and suffering from thyrotoxicosis (over-functioning of the thyroid gland) may also result in symptoms of palpitation, fatigue, chest pain and shortness of breath. These diseases must be excluded before labelling a person as a heart patient.

for various body functions including maintenance of the integrity of the inner lining of blood vessels (endothelium). It is through the effect of nitric oxide at the molecular level that the drug Viagra used for sexual potency, works. Physical exercise is thus also a good aphrodisiac and without any side-effects.

Q. What are the causes and cure for palpitation?

A. Palpitation is an uncomfortable awareness of the heartbeat. Normally one is not aware of one's heartbeat except during severe physical exercise or when under sudden emotional stress, or during sudden pressure like going for an interview or getting ready to ask a question from the speaker during a lecture. It is a manifestation of a fastly beating heart which may be regular or irregular. Palpitation is one of the four cardinal symptoms of heart disease, the other three being shortness of breath, chest pain and fatigue. Although palpitation may occur in any of the known structural heart diseases like rheumatic heart disease, congenital heart disease and coronary heart disease, it may also be present in a structurally normal heart. Palpitation starting suddenly and also ending abruptly is called Paroxymal Supraventricular Tachycardia (PSVT) and often occurs in otherwise normal hearts. Although there is a drug treatment for this condition, these days it can be permanently cured by a technique called Radiofrequency Ablation (RFA). Anaemia and thyroid disease, excessive tea, coffee, colas and alcohol can also cause palpitation.

Q. How harmful is cholesterol and how safe are cholesterol-lowering drugs? Are there any non-drug measures for lowering cholesterol?

A. Cholesterol is an important constituent of nerve cells and hormones, including sex hormones, and this is essential for our well-being. Beyond certain levels, however, generally above 200 mg/dl of blood and specially its subfraction LDL (Low Density Lipoprotein) beyond 100 mg/dl, it has been found to be a major risk factor for heart attacks. Its main source is food of animal origin like milk and dairy products and meats. Vegetables, fruits and nuts have no cholesterol. Apart from its exogenous source from food, cholesterol is also manufactured by our body, specially the liver, from other constituents of our diet. Taking a diet low in cholesterol and doing regular physical exercise do help to lower blood cholesterol to some extent. There are effective drugs available now to lower cholesterol, currently in vogue being **STATINS** like Lovastatin, Pravastatin and Simvastatin. The latest to appear in the market is Atorvastatin. They all help in lowering serum cholesterol to variable degrees with minimal side-effects. When taking these drugs one should periodically get blood tests carried out to look for any side-effects like muscle weakness and blood counts. Dosage may be adusted to keep total cholesterol between 150 to 200 mg and LDL below 100 mg.

Q. How does Echocardiography help in the diagnosis of the cause of chest pain?

A. Although, at present the Echo Test cannot detect the narrowing of coronary arteries throughout their length, but indirectly it can detect

Q. What is the difference between Stress Thallium Test and Tread Mill Test (TMT)?

A. Both these tests are used to diagnose the presence of ischaemic heart disease (ischaemia means lack of blood supply) which is the result of narrowing of coronary arteries (coronary artery disease). The Tread Mill Test (TMT) or cycle ergometery test as it is popularly known in most European countries is done when a patient complains of chest pain but his resting ECG shows no abnormality. During the test when the patient is made to run on a tread mill or do stationary cycling, if there are any ECG abnormalities, or

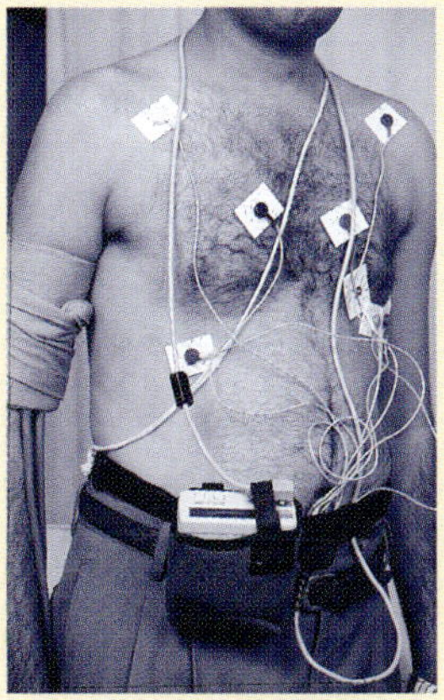

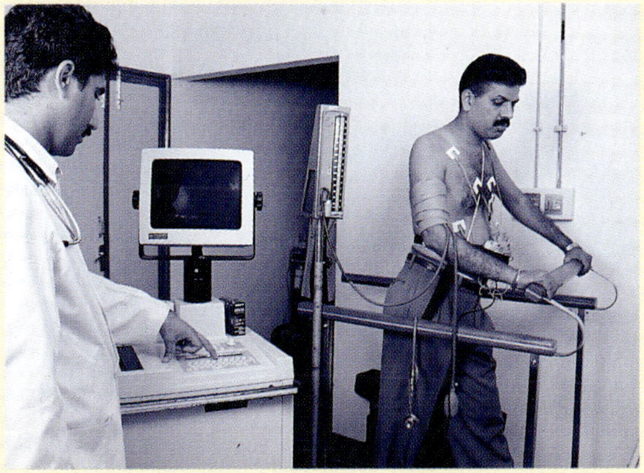

abnormal blood pressure response or the patient complains of angina, these findings help us in making the correct diagnosis of underlying coronary artery disease.

The Stess Thallium Test, on the other hand, is carried out by injecting a radioisotope material during exercise (cycle or tread mill) or after injecting a drug (dobutamine) and recording the distribution of blood flow to the various segments of heart muscle. This test helps to indicate the territorial distribution of the underlying coronary artery disease.

the wall motion abormalities in the heart muscle. Echo is helpful in the initial diagnosis of coronary events like angina or myocardial infarction (heart attack), it also helps subsequently in knowing whether the patient is improving or worsening. Hopefully the echo machines of the future will be able to detect the extent of actual narrowing in the blood vessels that supply blood to the heart muscle, thus giving us direct evidence of coronary artery disease. Presently the echo test is very useful in the diagnosis of other heart diseases like defects due to congenital and rheumatic heart disease.

Q. With the availability of CT scans and Magnetic Resonance Imagery (MRI) can one be saved from angiography?

A. Ultrasound CT scan helps in picking up calcium deposits in coronary arteries which suggest the strong possibility of the presence of coronary artery disease but not the extent of narrowing for which coronary angiography is still the gold standard. MRI done with the injection of a small amount of contrast medium (MR Angio) gives us some idea of disease in the major coronary arteries but as of now, when details of the entire coronary system are required to make decisions for bypass surgery or balloon angioplasty, a coronary angiography is still needed.

Q. What precautions should one observe while taking blood pressure-lower medicines?

A. When starting any anti-hypertension drug for the first time, one should look out for an undue fall in pressure as an individual response, especially on standing (postural hypotension). This is specially common in the elderly and among diabetics, so adequate instructions should be given to patients taking these drugs to avoid a sudden change in posture (standing erect from lying down) and if it frequently happens, medication should be changed under medical supervision. Fatigue, dry cough, impaired libido and impotence are some of the uncommonly observed side-effects of some anti-hypertensive drugs, which when observed, should be mentioned to the treating doctor for suitable change of therapy. While taking long-term treatment, periodic blood tests should be done for Haemogram, blood counts, sugar, urea, uric acid, electrolytes (Na^+, K^+) and blood lipid profile (cholesterol, triglycerides) as these may get altered by prolonged use of some of the blood pressure-lowering medicines.

Q. What is the role of yoga in the treatment of heart attacks?

A. Yoga is a way of living a healthy life through diet control, physical exercise and meditation. It has a great role in prevention of disease and promotion of health. But once there is strong evidence of major obstruction to blood flow due to significant blocks in the coronary arteries, relying only on yoga without actually tackling blocked blood vessels with other available means like drugs, devices or surgery, may not be the desirable strategy of treatment. Yoga must be practised as a good lifestyle measure to keep healthy. Along with other medical measures and after interventions and surgery, it helps to avoid recurrence of disease and to decrease drug requirements.

Q. How can one prevent rheumatic fever?

A. Rheumatic fever is more prevalent in overcrowded places (schools, crowded residential areas) where there are chances of easy spreading of bacterial throat infections. The preventive measures against rheumatic fever and rheumatic heart disease include: (1) Early detection of bacterial sore throat and its proper treatment with antibiotics; (2) Improving the general hygiene of living conditions, including improvement in nutrition of children; (3) Once rheumatic heart disease has been diagnosed, regular use of long-acting penicillin injection (once in three weeks) or other suitable antibiotic is advised. If a person is allergic to penicillin, recurrence of a sore throat should be avoided to prevent reappearance of rheumatic fever, so that any further damage to the heart can be prevented.

* * *

In any dialogue on management of heart disease and high blood pressure, there cannot be an epilogue and there should not be one. We do not still know all the reasons why heart attacks occur and why in some people blood flows at abnormally high pressure, while in others, it continues to flow smoothly at lower levels even beyond the age of three score plus ten. Even the same drugs produce varying responses and side-effects from person to person. Why is it that after ballooning, in some patients the disease occurs again, while in others it does not? Why do the grafts after by-pass surgery get blocked again in some, while they remain patent forever in others? Eating the same food, why does one member of a family get a heart attack and others do not? What are the protective factors for a healthy heart and longevity?

Is a heart transplant or a mechanical heart the answer to heart disease or will it be gene therapy? With the human genome being analysed and the mystery of life being further understood, the shape of treatment of disease in general, including heart disease, will be totally different in the next two decades. But there will still be more questions and thus the dialogue will continue . . . .

Commonly Used Medical Terminology in Heart Care

ACE: Angiotensin Converting Enzyme—An enzyme required for genesis of angiotensin—a powerful blood vessel constrictor.

Aneurysm: Circumscribed dilation of an artery.

Angina: Cardiac chest pain.

Angiography: Radiography of vessels after the injection of a radiopaque solution.

Angioplasty: Reconstruction of a blood vessel by ballooning.

Angiotensin: A potent vasoconstrictor (blood vessel constrictor).

Anorexia: Diminished appetite or aversion to food.

Aortic Stenosis: Narrow aortic valve.

Arrhythmia: Irregular rhythm of the heart.

Arteriole: A terminal artery.

Asphyxia: Impaired or lack of exchange of oxygen and carbon dioxide.

Atherectomy: The removal of fatty deposit in a blood vessel.

Atherogenesis: Narrowing of arteries.

Atherosclerosis: Blocked arteries due to fat deposition.

Atherosclerotic Plaques: Fatty streaks.

Atrial Septal Defect: A hole in the partition between the upper two chambers (atria) of the heart.

Broncho-spasm: Constriction of air passages.

CABG: Coronary Artery Bypass Graft.

Carboxyhaemoglobin: A stable union of carbon monoxide with haemoglobin.

Carcinogenic: Cancer-producing substance.

Cardiomyopathy: Flabby heart muscle or heart muscle disease.

Cardiovascular: Relating to the heart and blood vessels.

Cerebrovascular: Relating to blood vessels of the brain.

Chemotherapy: Treatment of disease by use of chemical substances.

Cholesterol: One of the blood fats found in body tissues, including the blood.

Claudication Pain: Diminished blood supply to the limbs causing pain in the legs on walking.

Coronary Arterial Tone: A temporary narrowing of the blood vessels.

Coarctation: Congenital narrowing (of aorta).

Corpulmonale: Heart disease secondary to lung disease.

CT: Computerised Tomography (method of radiography displaying details in a selected plane of the body.

Cyanosis: Deficient oxygenation of the blood leading to a dark bluish or purplish coloration of the skin.

Digitalis: A drug to augment the heart function.

Diuretics: Drugs that result in frequent urination.

Endophrine: A substance akin to morphine.

Homeostasis: The state of equilibrium in the body with respect to various functions and chemical compositions of the fluids and tissues.

Hut Test: Head-up Tilt test—a test used for the diagnosis of syncope (fainting attacks).

Hyperinsulnemia: Excessive insulin in the blood.

Hypertension: High blood pressure.

Hypokalemia: An abnormally low concentration of potassium in the circulating blood.

Hyponatremia: An abnormally low concentration of sodium ions in the circulating blood.

Hypotension: Low blood pressure.

ICCU: Intensive Cardiac Care Unit

ICD: Implankable Cardioverter-Defibrillater—a device that helps in the prevention of sudden cardiac death due to heart rhythm abnormalities.

Leg Oedema: Swelling of the feet and legs.

Lipoprotein (LP): a risk factor blood fat for atherosclerosis.

Liver Cirrhosis: *A* disease of the liver leading to body swelling and internal bleeding.

MRI: Magnetic Resonance Imaging.

Myocardial Infarction: Heart attack.

Myocardial Revascularisation: Re-establishment of the blood supply to the heart.

Myocardium: The middle layer of the heart consisting of the cardiac muscle.

Neuro-humoral Activity: Activity related to the nervous system and the endocrine system.

Osteoarthritis: Degnerative joint disease.

PTMR: Percutaneous Trans-Myocardial Revascularisation — a method used to increase blood supply to the heart muscle through laser and other means.

Patent Ducts Arteriosus: Abnormal communication between the aorta (main blood vessel carrying pure blood to the whole body) and the pulmonary artery (main blood vessel carrying impure blood to the lungs).

Peripartum: Related to the period of pregnancy and delivery.

Prophylaxis: Prevention of disease.

Psychosomatic: Concerning the mind and body as a unit.

Pulmonary Oedema: Waterlogging in the lungs.

Radiotherapy: The use of particulate radiations in the treatment of disease.

Renal: Related to the kidneys.

Spironolactone: A useful drug in the treatment of congestive heart failure.

Splanchnic: Related to the abdominal organs.

Statins: Drugs that lower blood cholesterol and other harmful blood fats.

Stents: Small wire coils used to maintain normal blood flow in the ballooned blood vessels.

Syncope: Transitory loss of consciousness or blackouts.

Tachyarrhythmias: Rapid and, at times, irregular beating of the heart.

Triglycerides: Another blood fat like cholesterol.

Ultrasonography: The location, measurement or delineation of deep structures by ultrasonic waves.

VLDL: Very Low Density Lipoprotein: it carries blood triglycerides.

Valvoplasty: The opening of narrow stenotic valves.

Vasopasm: A temporary narrowing of blood vessels.

Ventricular Septal Defect: A hole in the partition between the lower (muscular) chambers (ventricles) of the heart.